ZERO - GLUTEN

150 Plus Easy Gluten Free Recipes

Dr. Gianna Evelyn

CONTENTS

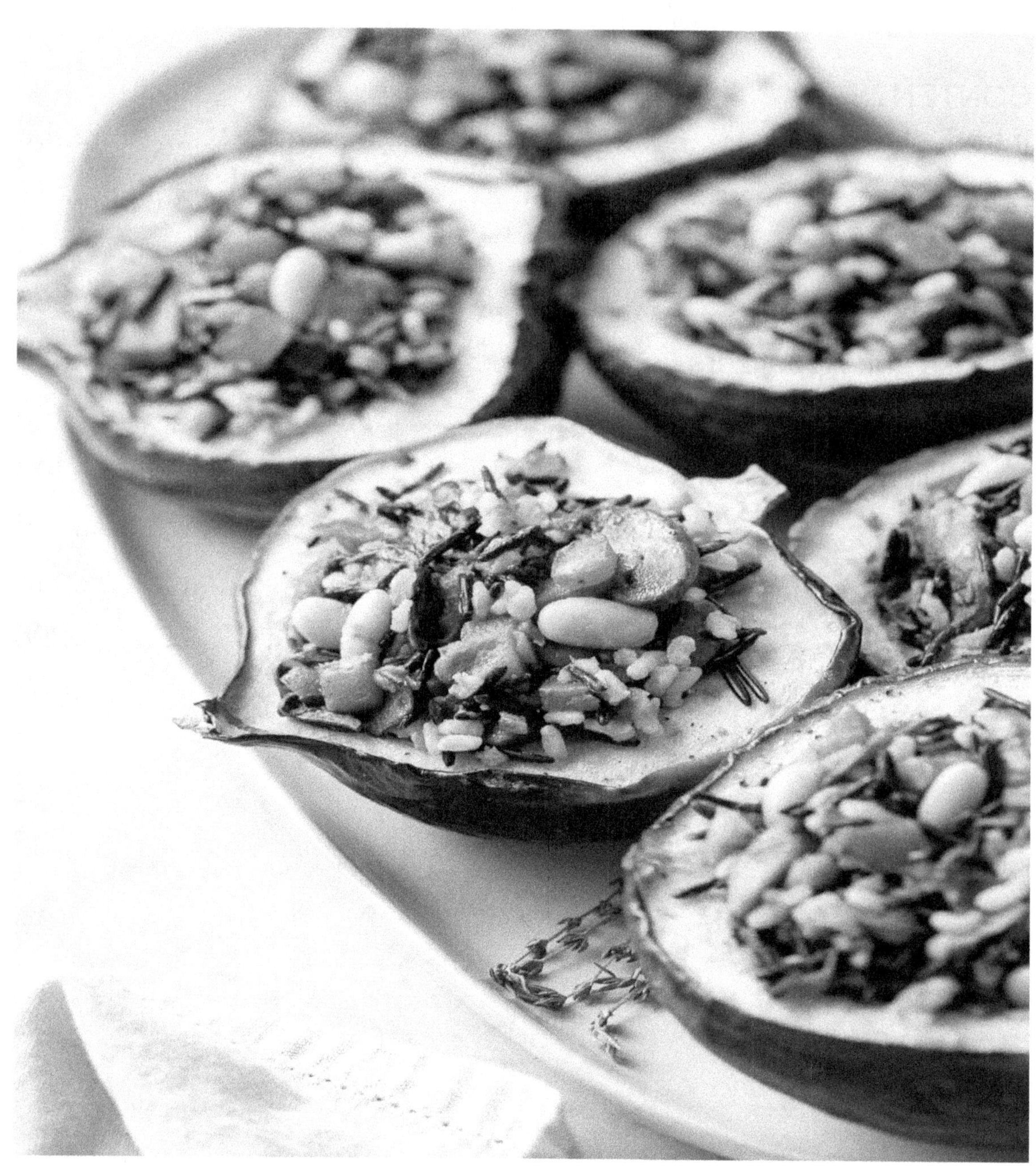

Introduction

What is Gluten?

Gluten is a protein complex primarily found in wheat, barley, and rye. It's responsible for the elastic texture of dough, allowing it to rise and maintain its shape, and provides a chewy texture to baked goods. Gluten is ubiquitous in many foods, not just in obvious items like bread and pasta, but also in sauces, dressings, and even some cosmetics and medications due to its binding properties.

Why Go Gluten-Free?

The decision to adopt a gluten-free diet can stem from various health-related reasons:

Celiac Disease: This autoimmune disorder is triggered by gluten. When individuals with celiac disease consume gluten, their immune system attacks the small intestine, leading to nutrient malabsorption and a wide range of symptoms, including digestive issues, anemia, and fatigue. The only treatment is a strict gluten-free diet.

Non-Celiac Gluten Sensitivity: Some people experience symptoms similar to those of celiac disease, such as bloating, gas, and abdominal pain, without the autoimmune intestinal damage. A gluten-free diet can alleviate these symptoms.

Wheat Allergy: Like other allergies, a wheat allergy involves an immune response to proteins found in wheat, including gluten. Avoiding gluten prevents allergic reactions.

Other Health Benefits: Many people report feeling better overall when they eliminate gluten from their diets. Benefits can include improved digestive health, increased energy levels, reduced inflammation, and a healthier diet overall.

The Gluten-Free Lifestyle

Living gluten-free involves more than avoiding bread and pasta. It's about being vigilant with food labels, understanding cross-contamination risks, and finding nutritious alternatives to gluten-containing grains. Gluten-free grains like quinoa, rice, and corn offer safe and healthy options.

Challenges and Considerations

While a gluten-free diet can be healthier for those with gluten-related disorders, it can also pose challenges, such as ensuring adequate intake of fiber and other nutrients typically found in whole-grain wheat products. It's important to balance the diet with a variety of foods to meet nutritional needs.

Whether due to medical necessity or personal choice, going gluten-free can lead to significant health improvements for many. It requires education, adaptation, and a commitment to maintaining a balanced diet, but the benefits for those sensitive to gluten can be life-changing.

Understanding Food Labels for a Gluten-Free Lifestyle

Navigating the world of gluten-free eating requires a keen eye for detail, especially when it comes to understanding food labels. Here's a comprehensive guide to help you make informed choices while shopping for gluten-free products.

1. The Gluten-Free Label

The most straightforward indicator of a gluten-free product is the "gluten-free" label. In many countries, including the United States, food products labeled as "gluten-free" must contain less than 20 parts per million (ppm) of gluten[1]. This strict standard ensures that the product is safe for individuals with celiac disease or gluten sensitivity.

2. Certification Marks

Look for certification marks from reputable organizations that verify the gluten-free status of a product. These certifications often involve rigorous testing and ensure that the product meets stringent gluten-free standards.

3. Ingredient List

Always read the ingredient list carefully. Ingredients derived from wheat, barley, rye, and oats (unless labeled gluten-free) should be avoided. Be aware of derivatives like malt (from barley) and hydrolyzed wheat protein, which also contain gluten.

4. Allergen Statement

The allergen statement, usually found near the ingredient list, will indicate if the product contains wheat, which is one of the top eight allergens required to be listed by law. However, a product may still be gluten-free if it contains wheat derivatives that have been processed to remove gluten, such as glucose syrup or maltodextrin from wheat[2].

5. Cross-Contamination Warnings

Some products may carry warnings such as "manufactured in a facility that also processes wheat." These warnings indicate a risk of cross-contamination, and while the product's ingredients are gluten-free, the presence of gluten cannot be guaranteed.

6. Decoding Uncertain Ingredients

If you encounter ingredients that are unclear, such as "natural flavors" or "modified food starch," it's best to contact the manufacturer for clarification on their gluten status.

7. Understanding 'Wheat-Free' vs. 'Gluten-Free'

"Wheat-free" does not necessarily mean "gluten-free." Wheat-free products may still contain gluten from other sources like barley or rye. Always look for the "gluten-free" label to be certain.

8. The Role of Technology

Utilize technology to your advantage. There are apps and websites dedicated to helping you identify gluten-free products and understand food labels better.

9. When in Doubt

If you're ever unsure about the gluten-free status of a product, it's safer to leave it on the shelf. Opt for whole, unprocessed foods like fruits, vegetables, and meats, which are naturally gluten-free and carry no risk of containing hidden gluten.

Benefits and Challenges of a Gluten-Free Diet

Embarking on a gluten-free diet can be a transformative experience, offering numerous benefits for those with gluten-related disorders and presenting unique challenges that require careful navigation.

Benefits of a Gluten-Free Diet

Alleviates Symptoms for Celiac Disease and Gluten Sensitivity: For individuals with celiac disease, a gluten-free diet is the only known treatment that can alleviate symptoms and prevent long-term complications. Similarly, those with non-celiac gluten sensitivity may find relief from chronic symptoms like abdominal pain, bloating, and fatigue.

Reduces Inflammation: Some people may experience a reduction in inflammation when removing gluten from their diet, which can lead to an overall feeling of improved health.

Promotes Nutrient Absorption: By healing the damaged intestinal lining in celiac disease patients, a gluten-free diet can improve nutrient absorption, leading to better overall health.

Encourages Whole Foods: A well-planned gluten-free diet often leads to an increased intake of whole, unprocessed foods such as fruits, vegetables, and lean proteins, contributing to a more balanced and nutritious diet.

May Improve Other Conditions: Some individuals report improvements in other health conditions, such as lactose intolerance, when they adopt a gluten-free diet.

Challenges of a Gluten-Free Diet

Risk of Nutritional Deficiencies: Without proper planning, a gluten-free diet can be low in fiber, iron, calcium, and B vitamins. It's important to ensure a balanced intake of nutrients, possibly with the help of supplements or fortified foods.

Limited Food Choices: Dining out or finding gluten-free options at social events can be challenging, as gluten is a common ingredient in many foods.

Potential for Unhealthy Substitutes: Many packaged gluten-free products are high in sugar, fat, and simple carbohydrates. It's crucial to make healthful choices and not just rely on processed gluten-free foods.

Cost: Gluten-free products often come with a higher price tag, which can make maintaining the diet more expensive.

Cross-Contamination Risks: For those with celiac disease, even small amounts of gluten can cause symptoms. Cross-contamination can occur in shared cooking environments, both at home and in restaurants.

A gluten-free diet can offer significant health benefits, particularly for those with celiac disease or gluten sensitivity. However, it also presents challenges that require attention to detail and careful planning. By focusing on whole, naturally gluten-free foods and being mindful of nutritional needs, one can navigate these challenges successfully. Always consult with a healthcare professional or a registered dietitian to ensure that your gluten-free diet is both safe and nutritionally adequate.

Breakfast

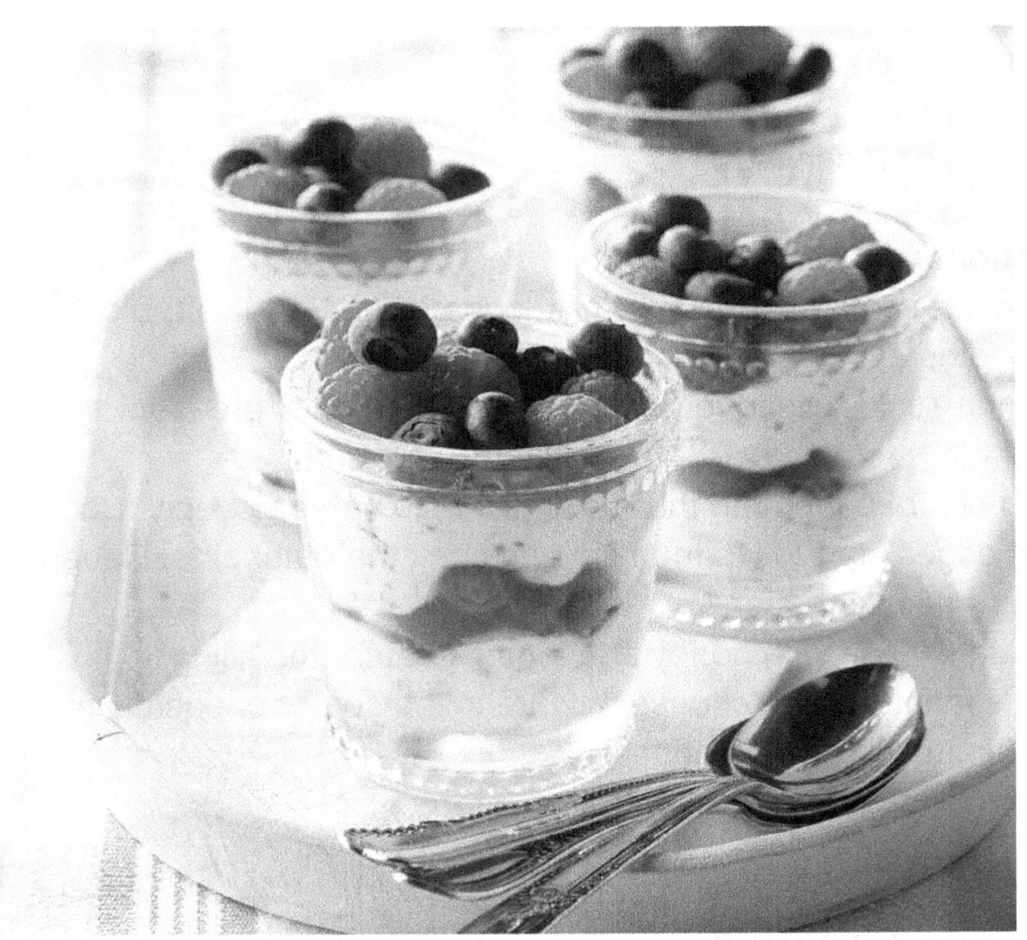

Gluten-Free Breakfast Blintzes
Ingredients:
1 cup gluten-free all-purpose flour
1 1/2 cups milk (dairy or non-dairy alternative)

2 large eggs
1 tablespoon sugar
1/4 teaspoon salt
Butter or oil for frying
1 cup ricotta cheese
1 tablespoon honey
Zest of 1 lemon
Fresh berries for serving

Instructions:
In a blender, combine the flour, milk, eggs, sugar, and salt. Blend until smooth.
Heat a non-stick skillet over medium heat and lightly grease with butter or oil.
Pour 1/4 cup of batter into the skillet, tilting to spread evenly. Cook until the edges start to lift, then flip and cook the other side. Repeat with the remaining batter.
Mix ricotta cheese with honey and lemon zest for the filling.
Place a spoonful of the cheese mixture in the center of each blintz and roll up, tucking in the edges.
Serve the blintzes with fresh berries on top.

Hash Brown Quiche Cups
Ingredients:
2 cups shredded potatoes (squeeze out excess moisture)
1/4 cup melted butter
Salt and pepper to taste
6 large eggs
1/2 cup milk (dairy or non-dairy alternative)

1/2 cup shredded cheddar cheese (or dairy-free alternative)
1/2 cup chopped spinach
1/4 cup diced red bell pepper
1/4 cup diced onion

Instructions:
Preheat your oven to 375°F (190°C) and grease a muffin tin.
Mix the shredded potatoes with melted butter, salt, and pepper.
Press the mixture into the bottom and up the sides of the muffin
cups.
Bake for 15 minutes until the edges are golden brown.
In a bowl, whisk together eggs and milk. Stir in cheese, spinach, bell
pepper, and onion.
Pour the egg mixture into the baked hash brown cups, filling each
one.
Bake for 20-25 minutes, or until the eggs are set.
Let them cool for a few minutes before removing from the muffin tin.

Lemon Chia Seed Parfait
Ingredients:
1/4 cup chia seeds
1 cup almond milk (or any non-dairy milk)
2 tablespoons maple syrup
1 teaspoon vanilla extract
Zest of 1 lemon
2 tablespoons lemon juice
1 cup gluten-free granola

1 cup mixed berries (strawberries, blueberries, raspberries)

Instructions:
In a bowl, mix together the chia seeds, almond milk, maple syrup, vanilla extract, lemon zest, and lemon juice.
Cover and refrigerate for at least 2 hours, or overnight, until it thickens into a pudding-like consistency.
To assemble the parfait, layer a spoonful of chia pudding at the bottom of a glass.
Add a layer of gluten-free granola followed by a layer of mixed berries.
Repeat the layers until the glass is filled, finishing with a layer of berries on top.
Garnish with a sprinkle of lemon zest and a drizzle of maple syrup.
Enjoy this tangy and nutritious Lemon Chia Seed Parfait as a delightful start to your day!

Gluten-Free Banana Pancakes
Ingredients:
2 ripe bananas, mashed
2 eggs
1/2 cup gluten-free oat flour
1/2 teaspoon baking powder
1/4 teaspoon cinnamon
1/8 teaspoon salt
Butter or coconut oil for cooking
Maple syrup and sliced bananas for serving

Instructions:

In a mixing bowl, combine the mashed bananas and eggs until well blended.

Add the oat flour, baking powder, cinnamon, and salt to the banana mixture and stir until just combined.

Heat a non-stick skillet over medium heat and grease with butter or coconut oil.

Pour 1/4 cup of batter for each pancake onto the skillet. Cook until bubbles form on the surface, then flip and cook until golden brown on the other side.

Serve the pancakes warm with a drizzle of maple syrup and additional banana slices on top.

Homemade Sage Sausage Patties
Ingredients:

1 pound ground pork
1 tablespoon fresh sage, finely chopped
2 teaspoons fresh thyme, finely chopped
1 teaspoon garlic powder
1 teaspoon onion powder
1/2 teaspoon smoked paprika
1/2 teaspoon black pepper
1/2 teaspoon sea salt
1/4 teaspoon cayenne pepper (optional)
1 tablespoon olive oil for cooking

Instructions:

In a large bowl, combine the ground pork with sage, thyme, garlic powder, onion powder, smoked paprika, black pepper, sea salt, and cayenne pepper.

Mix well until all the spices are evenly distributed throughout the meat.

Form the mixture into small patties, about 2 inches in diameter.

Heat olive oil in a skillet over medium heat.

Cook the patties for about 4-5 minutes on each side or until fully cooked and golden brown.

Serve hot and enjoy with your favorite gluten-free breakfast sides.

Farmer's Breakfast
Ingredients:
3 large potatoes, diced
1 small onion, diced
1 bell pepper, diced
6 eggs, beaten
1/2 cup shredded cheddar cheese (gluten-free)
4 strips of bacon, cooked and crumbled
2 tablespoons milk (dairy or non-dairy)
Salt and pepper to taste
2 tablespoons olive oil

Instructions:
In a large skillet, heat olive oil over medium heat.

Add the diced potatoes and cook until they start to soften, about 10 minutes.

Add the onions and bell peppers, and continue to cook until the vegetables are tender.

In a bowl, whisk together the eggs, milk, salt, and pepper.
Pour the egg mixture over the cooked vegetables in the skillet.
Sprinkle the shredded cheese and crumbled bacon on top.
Cover the skillet with a lid and let it cook until the eggs are set and
the cheese is melted, about 5-7 minutes.
Serve hot, garnished with fresh herbs if desired.

Zucchini Frittata
Ingredients:
2 medium zucchinis, thinly sliced
6 large eggs
1/2 cup milk (dairy or non-dairy)
1/2 cup grated Parmesan cheese (ensure it's gluten-free)
1/4 cup fresh basil, chopped
2 tablespoons olive oil
Salt and pepper to taste

Instructions:
Preheat your oven to 375°F (190°C).
In an oven-safe skillet, heat the olive oil over medium heat. Add the
zucchini slices and sauté until tender, about 5 minutes. Season with
salt and pepper.
In a bowl, whisk together the eggs, milk, Parmesan cheese, and
basil. Pour this mixture over the zucchini in the skillet.
Cook for 2-3 minutes until the edges begin to set.
Transfer the skillet to the oven and bake for 10-15 minutes, or until
the frittata is set and lightly golden on top.

Remove from the oven, let it cool slightly, and cut into wedges to serve.

Breakfast Skewers
Ingredients:
8 wooden skewers, soaked in water for 30 minutes
16 cherry tomatoes
8 button mushrooms, halved
1 bell pepper, cut into 1-inch pieces
1 large red onion, cut into wedges
8 slices of gluten-free ham, cut into 1-inch squares
2 tablespoons olive oil
Salt and pepper to taste
1 teaspoon dried oregano

Instructions:
Preheat your grill to medium-high heat.
Thread the tomatoes, mushrooms, bell pepper, onion, and ham onto the skewers, alternating between each ingredient.
Brush the skewers with olive oil and season with salt, pepper, and oregano.
Grill the skewers for 3-4 minutes on each side, or until the vegetables are tender and the ham is slightly charred.
Serve hot, perhaps with a side of gluten-free toast or a dollop of your favorite sauce.

Fresh Fruit Bowl
Ingredients:
1/2 cup watermelon, cubed
1/2 cup pineapple, cubed
1/2 cup papaya, cubed
1 kiwi, sliced
1/2 cup mango, cubed
1/2 cup strawberries, halved
1/4 cup blueberries
1/4 cup pomegranate seeds
Fresh mint leaves for garnish
Juice of 1 lime
1 tablespoon honey (optional)

Instructions:
In a large bowl, combine all the cubed and sliced fruits.
Drizzle with lime juice and honey, if using, and gently toss to coat the fruits.
Garnish with fresh mint leaves.
Chill in the refrigerator for at least 30 minutes before serving to allow the flavors to meld.
Serve in individual bowls and enjoy a refreshing start to your day

!

Veggie Omelette with Goat Cheese
Ingredients:
3 large eggs
1/4 cup milk (dairy or non-dairy)
Salt and pepper to taste

1/4 cup red bell pepper, diced
1/4 cup spinach, chopped
1/4 cup mushrooms, sliced
2 tablespoons goat cheese, crumbled
1 tablespoon olive oil or butter

Instructions:
In a bowl, whisk together the eggs, milk, salt, and pepper.
Heat the olive oil or butter in a non-stick skillet over medium heat.
Sauté the bell pepper, spinach, and mushrooms until they are just tender.
Pour the egg mixture over the vegetables in the skillet.
As the eggs begin to set, gently lift the edges with a spatula and tilt the pan to allow the uncooked eggs to flow underneath.
When the omelette is almost set, sprinkle the goat cheese over one half.
Carefully fold the omelette in half and cook for another minute or until the cheese begins to melt.
Slide the omelette onto a plate and serve hot.

Cranberry Banana Smoothie
Ingredients:
1 ripe banana
1/2 cup fresh or frozen cranberries
1/2 cup Greek yogurt (gluten-free)
1/2 cup orange juice
1 tablespoon honey or maple syrup
1/2 teaspoon vanilla extract

A pinch of cinnamon
Ice cubes (optional)

Instructions:
In a blender, combine the banana, cranberries, Greek yogurt, orange
juice, honey or maple syrup, vanilla extract, and cinnamon.
Blend until smooth. If the mixture is too thick, you can add a little
more orange juice to reach your desired consistency.
Add ice cubes if you prefer a colder smoothie and blend again.
Pour into a glass and garnish with a few cranberries on top for a
festive touch.
Enjoy this tangy and sweet smoothie as a quick and nutritious
breakfast option!

Protein-Rich Vegetable Quinoa Egg Muffins
Ingredients:
1 cup cooked quinoa (make sure it's cooled)
6 large eggs
1/4 cup milk (dairy or non-dairy)
1/2 cup chopped spinach
1/4 cup diced red bell pepper
1/4 cup diced onion
1/4 cup crumbled feta cheese (gluten-free)
Salt and pepper to taste
Cooking spray or oil for greasing

Instructions:

Preheat your oven to 350°F (175°C) and grease a muffin tin with cooking spray or oil.
In a large bowl, whisk together the eggs, milk, salt, and pepper.
Stir in the cooked quinoa, spinach, bell pepper, onion, and feta cheese until well combined.
Spoon the mixture into the muffin cups, filling each about 3/4 full.
Bake for 20-25 minutes, or until the tops are firm to the touch and the eggs are cooked through.
Allow the muffins to cool for a few minutes before removing them from the tin.

Avocado Toast with Poached Egg and Arugula
Ingredients:
2 slices of gluten-free bread
1 ripe avocado
2 eggs
1 cup arugula
1 tablespoon olive oil
1 teaspoon lemon juice
Salt and pepper to taste
Red pepper flakes (optional)
1 teaspoon white vinegar (for poaching eggs)

Instructions:
Toast the gluten-free bread slices to your preferred crispiness.
Mash the avocado in a bowl and season with salt, pepper, and lemon juice.
Spread the mashed avocado evenly on the toasted bread slices.

In a pot, bring water to a simmer and add white vinegar. Crack an egg into a small bowl and gently slide it into the simmering water. Poach for 3-4 minutes for a soft yolk or longer for a firmer yolk. Repeat with the second egg.

Place the poached eggs on top of the avocado toast.

Toss the arugula with olive oil, lemon juice, salt, and pepper. Top the toast with the seasoned arugula.

Sprinkle with red pepper flakes for a spicy kick.

Enjoy this nutritious and satisfying Avocado Toast with a perfect balance of flavors and textures!

Quick Gluten-Free Bagels
Ingredients:
1 1/2 cups gluten-free all-purpose flour
2 teaspoons baking powder
1/2 teaspoon salt
1 cup Greek yogurt (make sure it's gluten-free)
1 egg, beaten (for egg wash)
Optional toppings: sesame seeds, poppy seeds, dried garlic flakes, dried onion flakes

Instructions:
Preheat your oven to 375°F (190°C) and line a baking sheet with parchment paper.

In a bowl, mix the gluten-free flour, baking powder, and salt.

Add the Greek yogurt to the dry ingredients and mix until a dough forms.

Divide the dough into 4 equal parts and roll each part into a rope.
Join the ends to form a bagel shape.
Place the bagels on the prepared baking sheet.
Brush the tops with the beaten egg and sprinkle with your choice of toppings.
Bake for 20-25 minutes, or until golden brown.

Sweet Potato Toast with Avocado and Egg
Ingredients:
1 large sweet potato, sliced lengthwise into 1/4-inch thick slices
1 ripe avocado, mashed
2 eggs, fried or poached
Salt and pepper to taste
Red pepper flakes (optional)
Fresh cilantro or parsley for garnish

Instructions:
Toast the sweet potato slices in a toaster or toaster oven until they are tender and slightly crispy, usually about 2-3 cycles depending on your toaster.
Season the mashed avocado with salt and pepper, then spread it onto the sweet potato slices.
Top each slice with a fried or poached egg.
Sprinkle with red pepper flakes for a bit of heat, if desired.
Garnish with fresh cilantro or parsley before serving.
Enjoy this nutritious and satisfying twist on traditional toast!
Almond Flour Waffles
Ingredients:

2 cups almond flour
1 tablespoon coconut sugar (or sweetener of choice)
1 teaspoon baking powder
1/4 teaspoon salt
3 eggs
1/3 cup unsweetened almond milk (or milk of choice)
1/4 cup melted coconut oil or butter
1 teaspoon vanilla extract

Instructions:
Preheat your waffle iron according to the manufacturer's instructions.
In a large bowl, whisk together the almond flour, coconut sugar, baking powder, and salt.
In another bowl, beat the eggs and then mix in the almond milk, melted coconut oil, and vanilla extract.
Add the wet ingredients to the dry ingredients and stir until well combined.
Grease the waffle iron with a little oil or butter to prevent sticking.
Pour the batter onto the waffle iron and cook until golden brown and crispy.
Serve hot with your favorite toppings such as fresh berries, maple syrup, or whipped cream.

Coconut Yogurt Parfait with Tropical Fruits
Ingredients:
1 cup coconut yogurt
1/2 cup pineapple, diced
1/2 cup mango, diced
1/4 cup kiwi, sliced

1/4 cup granola (gluten-free)
2 tablespoons shredded coconut
1 tablespoon honey or agave syrup
A few mint leaves for garnish

Instructions:
In a glass or jar, start by layering 1/4 cup of coconut yogurt at the bottom.
Add a layer of diced pineapple and mango.
Sprinkle a layer of gluten-free granola and shredded coconut.
Repeat the layers until all ingredients are used, finishing with a layer of fruits on top.
Drizzle with honey or agave syrup for added sweetness.
Garnish with mint leaves for a refreshing touch.
Enjoy this tropical Coconut Yogurt Parfait as a sweet and healthy breakfast or snack!

Buckwheat Porridge with Cinnamon Apples
Ingredients:
1 cup buckwheat groats
2 cups almond milk or water
1 apple, peeled and diced
1/2 teaspoon cinnamon
1 tablespoon maple syrup
A pinch of salt
Chopped nuts and seeds for topping

Instructions:

Rinse the buckwheat groats under cold water until the water runs clear.

In a saucepan, combine the buckwheat groats, almond milk or water, and a pinch of salt.

Bring to a boil, then reduce the heat to low and simmer for 10-15 minutes, or until the porridge is creamy.

While the porridge is cooking, sauté the diced apple in a separate pan with cinnamon and maple syrup until tender.

Serve the buckwheat porridge in bowls topped with the cinnamon apples.

Add a sprinkle of chopped nuts and seeds for texture and extra nutrition.

Chickpea Flour Pancakes

Ingredients:

1 cup chickpea flour (also known as gram flour or besan)
1 cup water
1/2 teaspoon turmeric powder
1/2 teaspoon cumin powder
1/4 teaspoon baking soda
Salt to taste
1/4 cup chopped fresh cilantro
1/4 cup finely chopped red onion
1 green chili, finely chopped (optional)
Olive oil for cooking

Instructions:

In a mixing bowl, whisk together the chickpea flour, water, turmeric, cumin, baking soda, and salt until smooth.
Stir in the chopped cilantro, red onion, and green chili if using.
Heat a non-stick pan over medium heat and brush with olive oil.
Pour a ladleful of batter onto the pan and spread it out to form a pancake.
Cook for 2-3 minutes on one side until bubbles form on the surface, then flip and cook for another 2 minutes until golden brown.
Repeat with the remaining batter.
Serve hot with your favorite gluten-free chutney or sauce.

Oatmeal with Fresh Berries
Ingredients:
1 cup gluten-free rolled oats
2 cups water or milk (dairy or non-dairy)
Pinch of salt
1/2 teaspoon vanilla extract
1 tablespoon maple syrup or honey
1/2 cup fresh berries (strawberries, blueberries, raspberries)
A sprinkle of chia seeds or flaxseeds (optional)

Instructions:
In a saucepan, bring the water or milk to a boil. Add the oats and a pinch of salt.
Reduce the heat to a simmer and cook the oats, stirring occasionally, for about 5 minutes or until they reach your desired consistency.
Remove from heat and stir in the vanilla extract and maple syrup or honey.

Serve the oatmeal in bowls and top with fresh berries.
Sprinkle with chia seeds or flaxseeds for an extra nutritional boost.

Egg and Spinach Breakfast Wraps
Ingredients:
4 large eggs
1 cup fresh spinach, chopped
1/4 cup feta cheese, crumbled
2 tablespoons milk (dairy or non-dairy)
Salt and pepper to taste
2 gluten-free tortillas
1 tablespoon olive oil
Optional toppings: sliced avocado, salsa, hot sauce

Instructions:
In a bowl, whisk together the eggs, milk, salt, and pepper.
Heat olive oil in a skillet over medium heat. Add the spinach and sauté until wilted.
Pour the egg mixture over the spinach and let it set for a few seconds. Then, gently scramble the eggs until they are just cooked through.
Sprinkle feta cheese over the eggs and remove from heat.
Warm the gluten-free tortillas in a separate pan or in the microwave.
Divide the egg and spinach mixture between the tortillas, add any optional toppings, and roll them up to form wraps.
Serve immediately for a warm, nutritious breakfast.
Chia Pudding with Mixed Berry Compote
Ingredients:
1/4 cup chia seeds

1 cup almond milk (or any non-dairy milk)
1 tablespoon maple syrup
1/2 teaspoon vanilla extract
1 cup mixed berries (fresh or frozen)
1 tablespoon water
1 teaspoon lemon juice
Additional maple syrup to taste

Instructions:
In a bowl, mix together the chia seeds, almond milk, maple syrup, and vanilla extract. Stir well to combine.
Cover and refrigerate for at least 4 hours, or overnight, until it thickens and becomes pudding-like.
For the compote, combine the mixed berries, water, and lemon juice in a saucepan. Cook over medium heat until the berries break down and the mixture thickens, about 10 minutes. Sweeten with additional maple syrup if desired.
To serve, layer the chia pudding and berry compote in glasses or bowls.
Enjoy this delightful and healthy chia pudding with a flavorful berry compote!

Gluten-Free Muesli
Ingredients:
2 cups gluten-free rolled oats
1/2 cup sliced almonds
1/2 cup pumpkin seeds
1/2 cup sunflower seeds

1/2 cup dried cranberries
1/2 cup raisins
1/4 cup flaxseeds
1/4 cup chia seeds
1 teaspoon cinnamon
A pinch of salt
Optional: 1/2 cup coconut flakes

Instructions:

In a large mixing bowl, combine the rolled oats, sliced almonds, pumpkin seeds, sunflower seeds, dried cranberries, raisins, flaxseeds, chia seeds, cinnamon, and salt.
If you're using coconut flakes, add them to the mix.
Stir all the ingredients until they are well combined.
Store the muesli in an airtight container at room temperature.
To serve, soak a portion of muesli in milk (dairy or non-dairy) or yogurt overnight in the refrigerator. In the morning, top with fresh fruits and a drizzle of honey or maple syrup if desired.
Enjoy this homemade gluten-free muesli that's both filling and energizing!

Quinoa Breakfast Bowl
Ingredients:
1 cup cooked quinoa (cooled)
1/2 cup almond milk (or any non-dairy milk)
1 tablespoon maple syrup
1/2 teaspoon vanilla extract
1/4 teaspoon cinnamon
1/4 cup blueberries
1/4 cup sliced strawberries

1 banana, sliced
2 tablespoons chopped nuts (almonds, walnuts, or pecans)
A sprinkle of hemp seeds or sesame seeds

Instructions:
In a bowl, mix the cooked quinoa with almond milk, maple syrup, vanilla extract, and cinnamon.
Heat the mixture in a saucepan over medium heat for a few minutes until warm, or microwave for 1-2 minutes.
Transfer the warm quinoa to a serving bowl.
Top the quinoa with blueberries, sliced strawberries, banana, and chopped nuts.
Sprinkle hemp seeds or sesame seeds on top for added texture and nutrition.
Serve immediately for a warm and hearty breakfast bowl.

Gluten-Free Crepes
Ingredients:
1 cup gluten-free all-purpose flour
1 1/2 cups milk (dairy or non-dairy alternative)
2 large eggs
2 tablespoons melted butter or coconut oil, plus extra for cooking
1 tablespoon sugar (optional for sweet crepes)
1/4 teaspoon salt
1/2 teaspoon vanilla extract (for sweet crepes)

Instructions:

In a blender, combine the flour, milk, eggs, melted butter or coconut oil, sugar (if making sweet crepes), salt, and vanilla extract. Blend until smooth.
Let the batter rest for 30 minutes at room temperature to allow the flour to absorb the liquid.
Heat a non-stick skillet over medium heat and lightly grease with butter or oil.
Pour about 1/4 cup of batter into the skillet, tilting to spread evenly. Cook for 1-2 minutes until the edges start to lift, then flip and cook the other side for another minute.
Repeat with the remaining batter, stacking the cooked crepes with wax paper in between to prevent sticking.
Serve the crepes filled with your choice of sweet or savory fillings such as fresh fruit, yogurt, jam, cheese, or ham.

Pumpkin Spice Smoothie
Ingredients:
1/2 cup pumpkin puree (canned or homemade)
1 ripe banana
1 cup almond milk (or any non-dairy milk)
1/2 teaspoon pumpkin pie spice
1 tablespoon maple syrup or honey
1/2 teaspoon vanilla extract
A pinch of salt
Ice cubes

Instructions:

In a blender, combine the pumpkin puree, banana, almond milk, pumpkin pie spice, maple syrup or honey, vanilla extract, salt, and ice cubes.
Blend until smooth and creamy.
Taste and adjust the sweetness or spices if needed.
Pour into a glass and sprinkle with a little extra pumpkin pie spice on top for garnish.

Gluten-Free Granola Bars
Ingredients:
2 cups gluten-free rolled oats
1/2 cup almond butter (or any nut butter of your choice)
1/2 cup honey or maple syrup
1/2 cup chopped almonds
1/4 cup pumpkin seeds
1/4 cup dried cranberries
1/4 cup dark chocolate chips (ensure they're gluten-free)
1 teaspoon vanilla extract
1/2 teaspoon cinnamon
A pinch of salt

Instructions:
Preheat your oven to 350°F (175°C) and line a baking pan with parchment paper.
In a large bowl, mix together the oats, almonds, pumpkin seeds, dried cranberries, chocolate chips, cinnamon, and salt.

In a small saucepan, warm the almond butter and honey or maple syrup over low heat until smooth and combined. Remove from heat and stir in the vanilla extract.

Pour the wet ingredients over the dry ingredients and mix well until everything is coated.

Transfer the mixture to the prepared baking pan and press down firmly into an even layer.

Bake for 20-25 minutes, or until the edges are golden brown.

Allow the bars to cool completely in the pan before cutting into bars or squares.

Enjoy these homemade gluten-free granola bars as a convenient and healthy snack!

Egg and Avocado Salad
Ingredients:
4 hard-boiled eggs, peeled and chopped
2 ripe avocados, diced
1/4 cup red onion, finely chopped
1 tablespoon fresh cilantro, chopped
Juice of 1 lime
2 tablespoons olive oil
Salt and pepper to taste
Mixed greens or lettuce leaves for serving

Instructions:
In a medium bowl, gently combine the chopped eggs, diced avocados, red onion, and cilantro.

Drizzle with lime juice and olive oil, then season with salt and pepper.
Toss the salad gently to mix without mashing the avocado.
Serve the egg and avocado salad over a bed of mixed greens or lettuce leaves.

Berry and Yogurt Smoothie
Ingredients:
1 cup mixed berries (strawberries, blueberries, raspberries, blackberries)
3/4 cup Greek yogurt (ensure it's gluten-free)
1/2 cup almond milk (or any non-dairy milk)
1 tablespoon honey or maple syrup
1 teaspoon chia seeds
A few ice cubes

Instructions:
In a blender, combine the mixed berries, Greek yogurt, almond milk, honey or maple syrup, and chia seeds.
Add ice cubes to the blender for a chilled smoothie.
Blend on high speed until smooth and creamy.
Taste and adjust sweetness if necessary.
Pour into a glass and enjoy immediately.
This Berry and Yogurt Smoothie is a refreshing and nutritious way to start your day or as a midday pick-me-up!

Gluten-Free Cornbread
Ingredients:

1 cup gluten-free cornmeal
1 cup gluten-free all-purpose flour
1/4 cup sugar
1 tablespoon baking powder
1/2 teaspoon salt
1 cup milk (dairy or non-dairy)
1/3 cup melted butter or oil
2 large eggs

Instructions:
Preheat your oven to 400°F (200°C) and grease an 8-inch square baking pan.
In a large bowl, whisk together the cornmeal, flour, sugar, baking powder, and salt.
In another bowl, beat the milk, melted butter or oil, and eggs.
Add the wet ingredients to the dry ingredients and stir until just combined.
Pour the batter into the prepared pan and smooth the top.
Bake for 20-25 minutes, or until a toothpick inserted into the center comes out clean.
Let the cornbread cool slightly before cutting into squares and serving.

Breads and Pastries

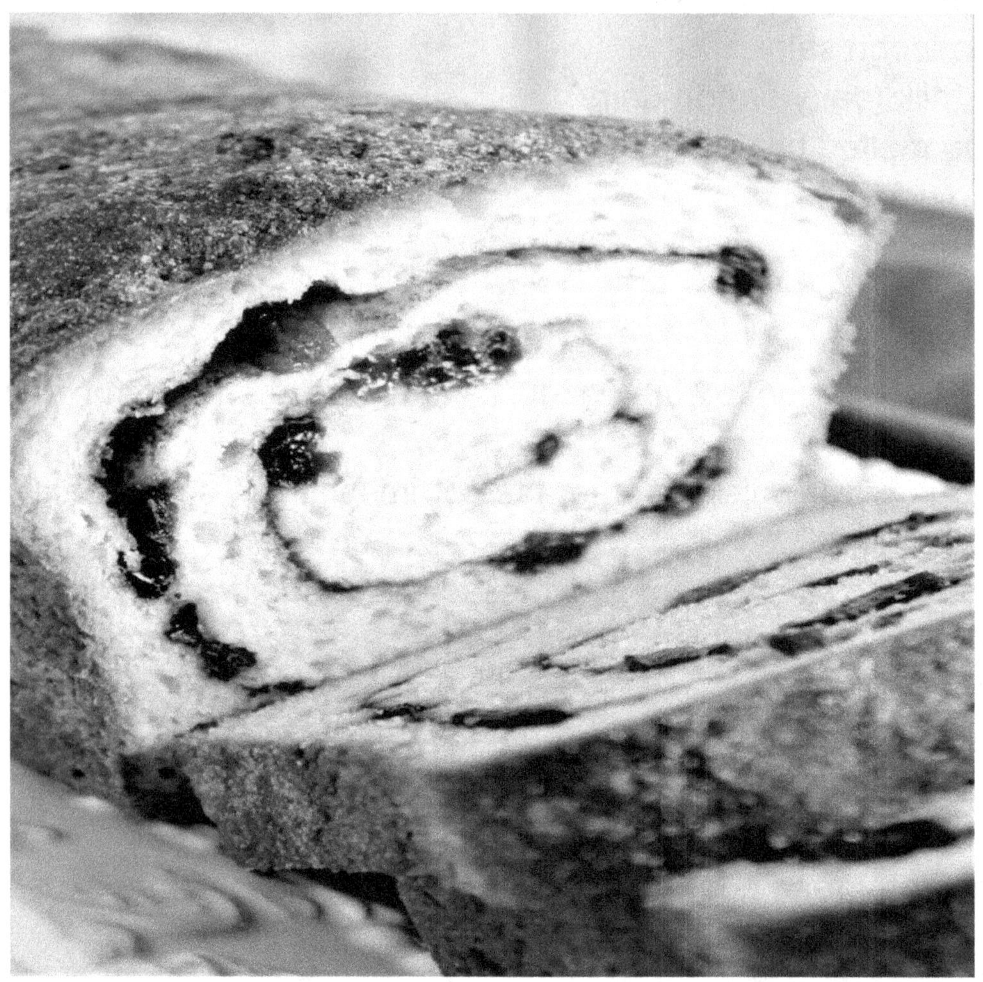

Crusty Artisan Gluten-Free Bread
Ingredients:
1 ½ cups warm water (110°F)
2 tsp sugar

1 tbsp instant yeast
3 cups gluten-free flour blend
1 ½ tsp salt
2 tbsp olive oil
1 tbsp apple cider vinegar
¼ cup psyllium husk powder

Instructions:
In a large bowl, dissolve sugar in warm water. Sprinkle yeast over the top and let stand for 5 minutes until foamy.
Add the gluten-free flour blend, salt, olive oil, apple cider vinegar, and psyllium husk powder to the yeast mixture. Stir until well combined.
Transfer the dough to a floured surface and knead for 5 minutes. The dough should be slightly sticky but manageable.
Shape the dough into a round loaf and place it on a baking sheet lined with parchment paper.
Cover with a damp cloth and let rise in a warm place for 1 hour, or until doubled in size.
Preheat your oven to 450°F (230°C). Place a pan of water on the bottom rack to create steam.
Once risen, slash the top of the loaf with a sharp knife to create a pattern.
Bake for 35-40 minutes, or until the bread is golden brown and sounds hollow when tapped on the bottom.
Remove from the oven and let cool on a wire rack before slicing.

Everyday Gluten-Free Loaf
Ingredients:
2 cups gluten-free flour blend

1 tbsp instant yeast
1 tsp sugar
1 tsp salt
1 ¼ cups warm milk (110°F)
2 eggs
2 tbsp vegetable oil
Instructions:
In a large bowl, combine the gluten-free flour blend, yeast, sugar, and salt.
In a separate bowl, whisk together the warm milk, eggs, and vegetable oil.
Add the wet ingredients to the dry ingredients and mix until a sticky dough forms.
Transfer the dough to a greased 9x5 inch loaf pan and smooth the top with a wet spatula.
Cover with a damp cloth and let rise in a warm place for 30 minutes, or until the dough has risen to the top of the pan.
Preheat your oven to 375°F (190°C).
Bake for 35-40 minutes, or until the top is golden brown and a toothpick inserted into the center comes out clean.
Remove from the oven and let cool in the pan for 10 minutes, then transfer to a wire rack to cool completely.

Hearty Multigrain Gluten-Free Bread
Ingredients:
1 cup warm water
2 tsp honey
1 tbsp instant yeast
1 cup gluten-free all-purpose flour

1 cup gluten-free multigrain flour mix
1/4 cup rolled oats
1/4 cup buckwheat groats
2 tbsp flaxseed meal
2 tbsp chia seeds
1/4 cup sunflower seeds
1/4 cup pumpkin seeds
1 tsp salt
2 tbsp olive oil
1 tbsp apple cider vinegar
2 tsp psyllium husk powder
Instructions:
Preheat your oven to 350°F (175°C). In a large bowl, dissolve honey in warm water, then sprinkle yeast over the top. Let it sit for 5 minutes until it becomes frothy.

In a separate bowl, mix together the gluten-free flours, oats, buckwheat, flaxseed meal, chia seeds, sunflower seeds, pumpkin seeds, and salt.

To the yeast mixture, add olive oil, apple cider vinegar, and psyllium husk powder. Stir well.

Gradually add the dry ingredients to the wet, mixing until a dough forms.

Transfer the dough to a greased loaf pan and smooth the top with a wet spatula.

Cover with a damp cloth and let it rise in a warm place for 30 minutes.

Bake for 40-45 minutes, or until the bread is golden brown and sounds hollow when tapped.

Let it cool before slicing. Enjoy your hearty, seed-filled bread!

Cinnamon Raisin Swirl Gluten-Free Bread

Ingredients:

1 1/2 cups gluten-free all-purpose flour

1/2 cup almond flour

2 tsp baking powder

1/2 tsp salt

1 tbsp instant yeast

1 cup warm milk

1/4 cup unsalted butter, melted

1/4 cup honey

1 egg

1/2 cup raisins

2 tbsp cinnamon

1/4 cup brown sugar

Instructions:

Preheat your oven to 375°F (190°C). In a bowl, combine the gluten-free flour, almond flour, baking powder, salt, and yeast.

In another bowl, whisk together warm milk, melted butter, honey, and the egg.

Add the wet ingredients to the dry ingredients and mix until just combined. Fold in the raisins.

Pour half of the batter into a greased loaf pan.

Mix together cinnamon and brown sugar, and sprinkle half over the batter in the pan.

Pour the remaining batter on top, and finish with the rest of the cinnamon-sugar mixture. Use a knife to swirl the cinnamon-sugar through the batter.

Bake for 30-35 minutes, or until a toothpick inserted into the center comes out clean.

Allow the bread to cool before slicing. Serve and enjoy your sweet, swirled treat!

Gluten-Free Rosemary Focaccia
Ingredients:
2 cups gluten-free flour blend
1 tbsp instant yeast
1 tsp sugar
1 ½ tsp salt
1 ½ cups warm water (110°F)
¼ cup extra virgin olive oil, plus more for drizzling
1 tbsp fresh rosemary, chopped
Coarse sea salt, for sprinkling
Instructions:
In a large mixing bowl, whisk together the gluten-free flour blend, instant yeast, sugar, and salt.
Add the warm water and ¼ cup olive oil to the dry ingredients and mix until a sticky dough forms.
Cover the bowl with a damp cloth and let it rise in a warm place for 1 hour, or until doubled in size.
Preheat your oven to 400°F (200°C). Line a baking sheet with parchment paper and transfer the dough onto it, spreading it out to your desired thickness.
Dimple the dough with your fingertips and drizzle with additional olive oil. Sprinkle the chopped rosemary and coarse sea salt over the top.
Bake for 20-25 minutes, or until golden brown and deliciously crisp.
Let it cool slightly before cutting into pieces. Serve warm and enjoy!

Gluten-Free Pumpkin Seed Bread

Ingredients:
2 cups gluten-free all-purpose flour
1 tbsp ground flaxseed
1 tsp baking soda
1/2 tsp salt
1/4 cup raw pumpkin seeds, plus extra for topping
1/4 cup sunflower seeds
1/4 cup olive oil
1 cup water
2 tbsp maple syrup
1 tbsp apple cider vinegar
1 tsp dried rosemary (optional)
Instructions:
Preheat your oven to 350°F (175°C) and grease a 9x5 inch loaf pan.
In a large bowl, whisk together the flour, ground flaxseed, baking soda, and salt.
Stir in the pumpkin seeds and sunflower seeds.
In a separate bowl, mix the olive oil, water, maple syrup, and apple cider vinegar.
Add the wet ingredients to the dry ingredients and stir until just combined. If using, fold in the dried rosemary.
Pour the batter into the prepared loaf pan and sprinkle the top with additional pumpkin seeds.
Bake for 45-50 minutes, or until a toothpick inserted into the center comes out clean.
Let the bread cool in the pan for 10 minutes, then transfer to a wire rack to cool completely.

Gluten-Free Chocolate Chip Banana Bread
Ingredients:

3 ripe bananas, mashed

2 cups gluten-free all-purpose flour

1 tsp baking powder

1/2 tsp baking soda

1/4 tsp salt

1/2 cup unsalted butter, softened

3/4 cup brown sugar

2 large eggs

1 tsp vanilla extract

1 cup chocolate chips

Instructions:

Preheat your oven to 350°F (175°C) and line a 9x5 inch loaf pan with parchment paper.

In a bowl, combine the mashed bananas with the softened butter, brown sugar, eggs, and vanilla extract. Mix until well combined.

In another bowl, sift together the flour, baking powder, baking soda, and salt.

Gradually add the dry ingredients to the wet ingredients, stirring until just combined.

Fold in the chocolate chips.

Pour the batter into the prepared loaf pan and smooth the top with a spatula.

Bake for 50-60 minutes, or until a toothpick inserted into the center comes out clean.

Allow the bread to cool in the pan for about 15 minutes before transferring it to a wire rack to cool completely.

Gluten-Free Spinach and Feta Bread

Ingredients:

2 cups gluten-free all-purpose flour

1 tbsp granulated sugar

2 tsp baking powder
1/2 tsp baking soda
1/2 tsp salt
1 cup fresh spinach, finely chopped
1/2 cup feta cheese, crumbled
2 large eggs
1 cup buttermilk
1/4 cup olive oil
1 tsp apple cider vinegar
1 tbsp fresh dill, chopped (optional)
Instructions:
Preheat your oven to 350°F (175°C) and grease a 9x5 inch loaf pan.
In a large bowl, whisk together the gluten-free flour, sugar, baking
powder, baking soda, and salt.
Stir in the chopped spinach and crumbled feta cheese until they are
evenly distributed throughout the flour mixture.
In a separate bowl, beat the eggs and then mix in the buttermilk,
olive oil, and apple cider vinegar.
Pour the wet ingredients into the dry ingredients and stir until just
combined. If using, fold in the chopped dill.
Transfer the batter to the prepared loaf pan and smooth the top with
a spatula.
Bake for 45-50 minutes, or until a toothpick inserted into the center
comes out clean.
Allow the bread to cool in the pan for 10 minutes before transferring
it to a wire rack to cool completely.

Gluten-Free Lemon Poppy Seed Loaf
Ingredients:
2 cups gluten-free all-purpose flour

1 tbsp baking powder
1/2 tsp salt
1/4 cup poppy seeds
Zest of 2 lemons
1/2 cup unsalted butter, softened
1 cup granulated sugar
3 large eggs
1/2 cup milk (dairy or non-dairy)
1/4 cup fresh lemon juice
1 tsp vanilla extract
Lemon Glaze:
1/2 cup powdered sugar
1 tbsp lemon juice
Instructions:
Preheat your oven to 350°F (175°C) and grease a 9x5 inch loaf pan.
In a bowl, whisk together the gluten-free flour, baking powder, salt,
and poppy seeds.
In another bowl, cream the butter, sugar, and lemon zest until light
and fluffy.
Beat in the eggs one at a time, then stir in the milk, lemon juice, and
vanilla extract.
Gradually mix the dry ingredients into the wet until just combined.
Pour the batter into the prepared loaf pan and bake for 50-60
minutes, or until a toothpick inserted into the center comes out clean.
For the glaze, whisk together the powdered sugar and lemon juice
until smooth. Drizzle over the cooled loaf.

Gluten-Free Cheddar Jalapeño Bread
Ingredients:
2 cups gluten-free all-purpose flour

1 tbsp sugar
2 tsp baking powder
1/2 tsp baking soda
1/2 tsp salt
1 cup sharp cheddar cheese, shredded
1/4 cup jalapeños, finely chopped (seeds removed for less heat)
1 cup buttermilk (or milk with 1 tbsp vinegar)
1/4 cup unsalted butter, melted
2 large eggs
Instructions:
Preheat your oven to 350°F (175°C) and grease a 9x5 inch loaf pan.
In a large bowl, combine the flour, sugar, baking powder, baking soda, and salt.
Stir in the shredded cheddar cheese and chopped jalapeños.
In another bowl, whisk together the buttermilk, melted butter, and eggs.
Add the wet ingredients to the dry ingredients and stir until just combined.
Pour the batter into the prepared loaf pan and bake for 45-50 minutes, or until a toothpick inserted into the center comes out clean.
Let the bread cool in the pan for 10 minutes before transferring to a wire rack to cool completely.

Gluten-Free French Croissants
Ingredients:
2 cups gluten-free all-purpose flour
1 tbsp granulated sugar
1 tsp salt
1 tbsp instant yeast
1/2 cup warm water

1/2 cup warm milk
1 cup unsalted butter, cold and cubed
1 egg, for egg wash
Instructions:
In a large bowl, mix together the flour, sugar, salt, and yeast.
Add the warm water and milk, and mix until a dough forms.
On a floured surface, roll out the dough into a rectangle. Distribute the butter cubes evenly over the dough, leaving a small border around the edges.
Fold the dough into thirds, like a letter, enclosing the butter. Turn the dough 90 degrees and roll it out again into a rectangle. Fold into thirds once more. Wrap in plastic and chill for 30 minutes.
Repeat the rolling and folding process two more times, chilling the dough for 30 minutes between each turn.
After the final chill, roll the dough out to a 1/4 inch thickness. Cut into triangles and roll each triangle tightly from the base to the tip to form a croissant shape.
Place the croissants on a baking sheet, cover loosely with plastic wrap, and let rise until doubled in size, about 1 hour.
Preheat the oven to 400°F (200°C). Brush the croissants with the beaten egg.
Bake for 15-20 minutes, or until golden brown. Cool on a wire rack before serving.

Gluten-Free Blueberry Lemon Muffins
Ingredients:
2 cups gluten-free all-purpose flour
1 tbsp baking powder
1/2 tsp salt
1 cup sugar

Zest of 1 lemon
1/2 cup unsalted butter, melted
2 large eggs
1 cup milk
1 tbsp lemon juice
1 tsp vanilla extract
1 1/2 cups fresh blueberries
Instructions:
Preheat your oven to 375°F (190°C) and line a muffin tin with paper liners.
In a large bowl, whisk together the flour, baking powder, salt, sugar, and lemon zest.
In a separate bowl, mix the melted butter, eggs, milk, lemon juice, and vanilla extract.
Add the wet ingredients to the dry ingredients and stir until just combined. Gently fold in the blueberries.
Divide the batter evenly among the muffin cups, filling each about 3/4 full.
Bake for 25-30 minutes, or until the muffins are golden and a toothpick inserted into the center comes out clean.
Let the muffins cool in the pan for 5 minutes, then transfer to a wire rack to cool completely.

Gluten-Free Lemon Poppy Seed Loaf
Ingredients:
2 cups gluten-free all-purpose flour
1 tbsp baking powder
1/2 tsp salt
3 tbsp poppy seeds
Zest of 2 lemons

3/4 cup granulated sugar

1/2 cup unsalted butter, softened

2 large eggs

1/2 cup Greek yogurt

1/4 cup fresh lemon juice

1 tsp vanilla extract

Lemon Glaze:

1 cup powdered sugar

2 tbsp lemon juice

Instructions:

Preheat your oven to 350°F (175°C) and grease a 9x5 inch loaf pan.

In a bowl, whisk together the gluten-free flour, baking powder, salt, and poppy seeds.

In a separate bowl, cream together the butter, sugar, and lemon zest until light and fluffy.

Beat in the eggs one at a time, then mix in the Greek yogurt, lemon juice, and vanilla extract.

Gradually add the dry ingredients to the wet, stirring until just combined.

Pour the batter into the prepared loaf pan and bake for 45-50 minutes, or until a toothpick inserted into the center comes out clean.

For the glaze, whisk together the powdered sugar and lemon juice until smooth. Drizzle over the cooled loaf.

Now, for the Cheddar Jalapeño Bread.

Gluten-Free Cheddar Jalapeño Bread

Ingredients:

2 cups gluten-free all-purpose flour

1 tbsp sugar

2 tsp baking powder

1/2 tsp baking soda

1/2 tsp salt
1 cup sharp cheddar cheese, shredded
1/4 cup jalapeños, finely chopped (seeds removed for less heat)
1 cup buttermilk
1/4 cup unsalted butter, melted
2 large eggs
Instructions:
Preheat your oven to 350°F (175°C) and grease a 9x5 inch loaf pan.
In a large bowl, combine the flour, sugar, baking powder, baking
soda, and salt.
Stir in the shredded cheddar cheese and chopped jalapeños.
In another bowl, whisk together the buttermilk, melted butter, and
eggs.
Add the wet ingredients to the dry ingredients and stir until just
combined.
Pour the batter into the prepared loaf pan and bake for 45-50
minutes, or until a toothpick inserted into the center comes out clean.
Let the bread cool in the pan for 10 minutes before transferring to a
wire rack to cool completely.

Gluten-Free Pecan Pumpkin Glazed Doughnuts

Ingredients:
1 1/2 cups gluten-free all-purpose flour
1/2 cup almond flour
1/4 cup granulated sugar
2 tsp baking powder
1/2 tsp salt
1 tsp cinnamon
1/2 tsp nutmeg
1/4 tsp cloves

1/4 tsp ginger
1 cup pumpkin purée
2 large eggs
1/4 cup vegetable oil
1/4 cup milk (dairy or non-dairy)
1/2 cup chopped pecans
Pumpkin Glaze:
1 cup powdered sugar
2 tbsp pumpkin purée
1/2 tsp vanilla extract
1-2 tbsp milk (as needed for consistency)
Instructions:
Preheat your oven to 350°F (175°C) and grease a doughnut pan.
In a large bowl, whisk together the gluten-free flour, almond flour, sugar, baking powder, salt, and spices.
In another bowl, mix the pumpkin purée, eggs, oil, and milk until smooth.
Add the wet ingredients to the dry ingredients and mix until just combined. Fold in the chopped pecans.
Spoon the batter into the doughnut pan, filling each cavity about 3/4 full.
Bake for 12-15 minutes, or until a toothpick comes out clean.
For the glaze, mix the powdered sugar, pumpkin purée, vanilla extract, and milk until smooth. Adjust the consistency with more milk if needed.
Once the doughnuts are cool, dip them into the glaze and let set on a wire rack.

Gluten-Free Coconut Banana Bread with Almond Streusel
Ingredients:

1 1/2 cups gluten-free all-purpose flour
1/2 cup coconut flour
1 tsp baking soda
1/2 tsp salt
4 ripe bananas, mashed
1/2 cup coconut oil, melted
3/4 cup brown sugar
2 large eggs
1 tsp vanilla extract
1/2 cup shredded coconut
Almond Streusel:
1/2 cup almond flour
1/4 cup brown sugar
1/4 cup cold butter, cubed
1/2 tsp cinnamon
1/4 cup sliced almonds
Instructions:
Preheat your oven to 350°F (175°C) and grease a 9x5 inch loaf pan.
In a bowl, combine the gluten-free flour, coconut flour, baking soda, and salt.
In a separate bowl, mix the mashed bananas, coconut oil, brown sugar, eggs, and vanilla extract.
Gradually add the dry ingredients to the wet, stirring until just combined. Fold in the shredded coconut.
Pour the batter into the prepared loaf pan.
For the streusel, mix the almond flour, brown sugar, and cinnamon in a bowl. Cut in the butter until the mixture resembles coarse crumbs. Stir in the sliced almonds.
Sprinkle the streusel over the batter in the loaf pan.

Bake for 50-60 minutes, or until a toothpick inserted into the center comes out clean.

Let the bread cool in the pan for 10 minutes before transferring to a wire rack to cool completely.

Gluten-Free Pumpkin Scones with Cinnamon Glaze

Ingredients:

2 cups gluten-free all-purpose flour

1/3 cup brown sugar

1 tbsp baking powder

1/2 tsp salt

1 tsp pumpkin pie spice

1/2 cup cold butter, cubed

1/2 cup pumpkin puree

1/4 cup heavy cream

1 large egg

1 tsp vanilla extract

Cinnamon Glaze:

1 cup powdered sugar

1/4 tsp cinnamon

2 tbsp milk

1/2 tsp vanilla extract

Instructions:

Preheat your oven to 425°F (220°C) and line a baking sheet with parchment paper.

In a large bowl, whisk together the flour, brown sugar, baking powder, salt, and pumpkin pie spice.

Cut in the cold butter until the mixture resembles coarse crumbs.

In a separate bowl, mix the pumpkin puree, heavy cream, egg, and vanilla extract.

Add the wet ingredients to the dry ingredients and stir until just combined.
Turn the dough out onto a floured surface and shape into a circle about 1 inch thick. Cut into 8 wedges.
Place the scones on the prepared baking sheet and bake for 14-16 minutes or until golden brown.
For the glaze, whisk together the powdered sugar, cinnamon, milk, and vanilla extract until smooth.
Drizzle the glaze over the warm scones and serve.

Gluten-Free Blueberry Buttermilk Breakfast Cake
Ingredients:
2 cups gluten-free all-purpose flour
3/4 cup sugar
2 tsp baking powder
1/2 tsp salt
Zest of 1 lemon
1/2 cup unsalted butter, softened
2 large eggs
1 tsp vanilla extract
1/2 cup buttermilk
1 1/2 cups fresh blueberries
Instructions:
Preheat your oven to 350°F (175°C) and grease a 9-inch round cake pan.
In a bowl, whisk together the flour, sugar, baking powder, salt, and lemon zest.
In another bowl, cream the butter until smooth. Add the eggs one at a time, then stir in the vanilla extract.

Alternately add the dry ingredients and buttermilk to the butter mixture, starting and ending with the dry ingredients.
Gently fold in the blueberries.
Pour the batter into the prepared pan and smooth the top.
Bake for 35-40 minutes or until a toothpick inserted into the center comes out clean.
Let the cake cool before serving. Optionally, dust with powdered sugar for a sweet finish.

Gluten-Free Savory Churro Waffles
Ingredients:
1 1/2 cups almond flour
1/2 tsp baking soda
1/2 tsp smoked paprika
1/4 tsp garlic powder
1/4 tsp onion powder
1/4 tsp salt
1/3 cup canned coconut milk
2 large eggs
1 tbsp olive oil
1/4 cup grated Parmesan cheese
1/4 cup shredded sharp cheddar cheese
2 tbsp chopped fresh chives
Instructions:
In a large bowl, mix together almond flour, baking soda, smoked paprika, garlic powder, onion powder, and salt.
Stir in coconut milk, eggs, and olive oil until well combined.
Fold in Parmesan cheese, cheddar cheese, and chives.
Preheat your waffle iron and grease it with a bit of olive oil.

Pour the batter into the waffle iron and cook according to the manufacturer's instructions until golden and crisp.
Serve hot with a dollop of sour cream or your favorite salsa.

Gluten-Free Apple Fritters
Ingredients:
1 1/2 cups gluten-free all-purpose flour
1/4 cup granulated sugar
2 tsp baking powder
1/2 tsp cinnamon
1/4 tsp nutmeg
1/4 tsp salt
2/3 cup milk (dairy or non-dairy)
2 large eggs, lightly beaten
1 tsp vanilla extract
2 cups diced apples
Vegetable oil for frying
Cinnamon Sugar Coating:
1/2 cup granulated sugar
1 tsp cinnamon
Instructions:
In a large bowl, whisk together the flour, sugar, baking powder, cinnamon, nutmeg, and salt.
Stir in the milk, eggs, and vanilla extract until the batter is smooth.
Fold in the diced apples.
Heat oil in a deep fryer or large pot to 375°F (190°C).
Carefully drop spoonfuls of the batter into the hot oil and fry for 2-3 minutes on each side, or until golden brown.
Remove the fritters with a slotted spoon and drain on paper towels.

Mix the sugar and cinnamon for the coating in a shallow dish. Roll the warm fritters in the cinnamon sugar to coat.
Serve warm and enjoy!

Gluten-Free Pear Tart
Ingredients:
1 1/2 cups gluten-free all-purpose flour
1/2 cup almond flour
1/4 cup granulated sugar
1/2 tsp salt
1/2 cup cold butter, cubed
4-6 Tbsp ice water
3 medium pears, ripe but still firm
1/2 cup brown sugar
2 tsp ground cinnamon
3 Tbsp lemon juice
Instructions:
In a food processor, pulse together gluten-free flour, almond flour, sugar, and salt.
Add cold butter and pulse until the mixture resembles coarse crumbs.
Gradually add ice water and pulse until the dough comes together.
Wrap the dough in plastic and chill for 30 minutes.
Preheat the oven to 375°F (190°C).
Roll out the dough and fit it into a 9-inch tart pan; trim the excess.
In a bowl, toss sliced pears with brown sugar, cinnamon, and lemon juice.
Arrange the pear slices in the tart shell in an overlapping pattern.
Bake for 45-50 minutes until the crust is golden and pears are tender.

Let cool before serving. Enjoy your gluten-free Pear Tart!
Now, for the Chocolate Tarts.

Gluten-Free Chocolate Tarts
Ingredients:
1 cup gluten-free all-purpose flour
1/4 cup cocoa powder
1/4 cup powdered sugar
1/2 tsp salt
1/2 cup cold butter, cubed
2-3 Tbsp cold water
1 cup heavy cream
8 oz dark chocolate, finely chopped
1 tsp vanilla extract

Instructions:
For the crust, mix flour, cocoa powder, powdered sugar, and salt.
Cut in butter until the mixture resembles coarse crumbs.
Add water and mix until a dough forms.
Press the dough into tart pans and refrigerate for 30 minutes.
Preheat the oven to 350°F (175°C).
Bake the crusts for 10-12 minutes. Let them cool.
For the filling, heat the cream until it just begins to simmer.
Pour over the chopped chocolate and let sit for 1 minute, then stir until smooth.
Stir in vanilla extract.
Pour the ganache into the cooled tart shells and refrigerate until set, about 2 hours.
Serve your Chocolate Tarts with a dusting of powdered sugar or a dollop of whipped cream.

Savory Spinach and Feta Gluten-Free Bread

Ingredients:

2 cups gluten-free all-purpose flour

1 tbsp granulated sugar

2 tsp baking powder

1/2 tsp baking soda

1/2 tsp salt

1 cup fresh spinach, finely chopped

1/2 cup feta cheese, crumbled

2 large eggs

1 cup buttermilk

1/4 cup olive oil

1 tsp apple cider vinegar

1 tbsp fresh dill, chopped (optional)

Instructions:

Preheat your oven to 350°F (175°C) and grease a 9x5 inch loaf pan.

In a large bowl, whisk together the gluten-free flour, sugar, baking powder, baking soda, and salt.

Stir in the chopped spinach and crumbled feta cheese until they are evenly distributed throughout the flour mixture.

In a separate bowl, beat the eggs and then mix in the buttermilk, olive oil, and apple cider vinegar.

Pour the wet ingredients into the dry ingredients and stir until just combined. If using, fold in the chopped dill.

Transfer the batter to the prepared loaf pan and smooth the top with a spatula.

Bake for 45-50 minutes, or until a toothpick inserted into the center comes out clean.

Allow the bread to cool in the pan for 10 minutes before transferring it to a wire rack to cool completely.

Soups and Salads

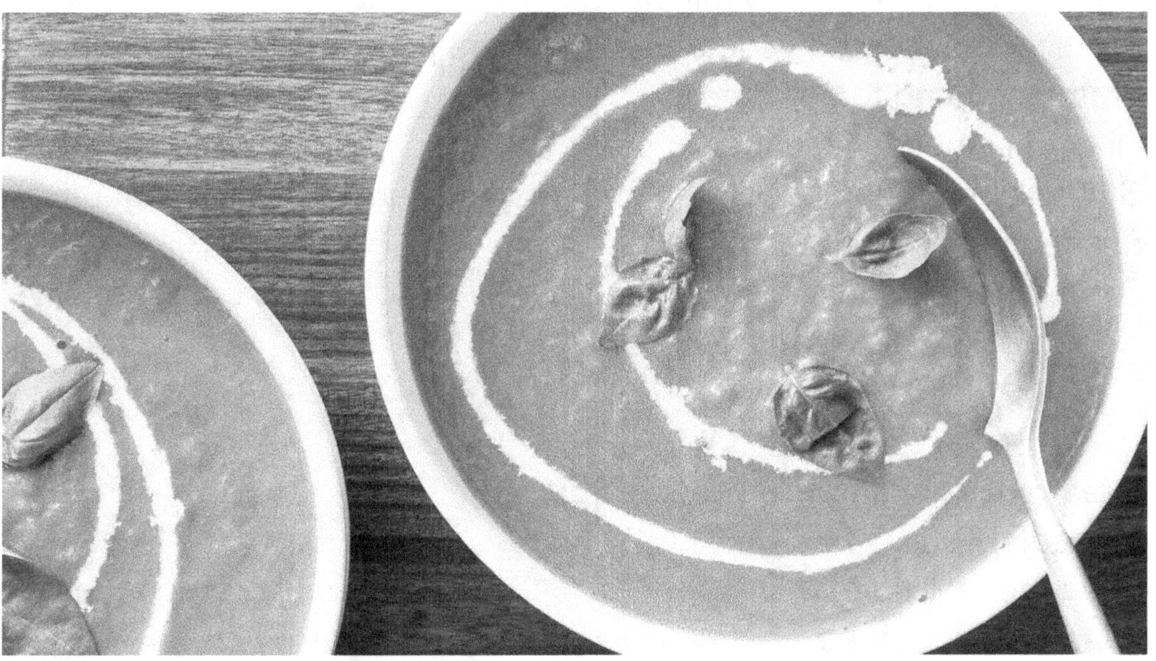

Classic Tomato Soup

Ingredients:

1 kg ripe tomatoes, quartered

2 medium onions, chopped

4 cloves garlic, minced

2 tbsp olive oil

1 tbsp balsamic vinegar

2 cups gluten-free vegetable broth

1/2 cup fresh basil leaves, chopped

Salt and pepper to taste

A pinch of sugar (optional)

Instructions:

Preheat your oven to 200°C (400°F). Place the tomatoes, onions, and garlic on a baking sheet and drizzle with olive oil and balsamic vinegar. Roast for 25-30 minutes until caramelized.
Transfer the roasted vegetables to a large pot. Add the vegetable broth and bring to a simmer.
Use an immersion blender to puree the soup until smooth.
Stir in the chopped basil, salt, and pepper. Add a pinch of sugar if desired to balance the acidity.
Simmer for an additional 10 minutes. Serve hot with a drizzle of olive oil or a dollop of gluten-free sour cream.

Creamy Broccoli and Cheese Soup
Ingredients:
500g broccoli florets
1 large carrot, diced
1 medium onion, diced
3 cups gluten-free chicken or vegetable broth
1 cup heavy cream
2 cups shredded cheddar cheese (ensure it's gluten-free)
2 tbsp gluten-free all-purpose flour
2 tbsp unsalted butter
Salt and pepper to taste
A pinch of nutmeg (optional)
Instructions:
In a large pot, melt the butter over medium heat. Add the onion and carrot, cooking until softened, about 5 minutes.
Sprinkle the flour over the vegetables and stir to coat. Cook for another minute.

Slowly add the broth while stirring continuously to avoid lumps. Bring to a boil.

Add the broccoli florets and reduce the heat. Simmer until the broccoli is tender, about 10 minutes.

Blend the soup with an immersion blender to your desired consistency.

Stir in the heavy cream and bring the soup back to a simmer.

Gradually add the shredded cheese, stirring until melted and smooth. Season with salt, pepper, and a pinch of nutmeg.

Serve warm with extra cheese on top if desired.

Chicken Noodle Soup

Ingredients:

2 tablespoons olive oil

1 pound chicken breast, cut into bite-sized pieces

1 medium onion, chopped

2 carrots, peeled and sliced

2 celery stalks, sliced

3 cloves garlic, minced

6 cups gluten-free chicken broth

2 bay leaves

1/2 teaspoon dried thyme

1/2 teaspoon dried oregano

2 cups gluten-free noodles

Salt and pepper to taste

Fresh parsley for garnish

Instructions:

Heat the olive oil in a large pot over medium-high heat. Add the chicken pieces and cook until browned. Remove the chicken and set aside.

In the same pot, add the onion, carrots, and celery. Cook until the vegetables are softened, about 5 minutes.
Add the garlic, bay leaves, thyme, and oregano. Cook for another minute until the garlic is fragrant.
Pour in the chicken broth and bring to a boil. Add the noodles and the cooked chicken.
Reduce the heat and simmer until the noodles are tender and the chicken is cooked through, about 10 minutes.
Season with salt and pepper to taste. Remove the bay leaves.
Serve hot, garnished with fresh parsley.

Minestrone Soup
Ingredients:
2 tbsp olive oil
1 medium onion, diced
2 carrots, peeled and diced
2 stalks celery, diced
3 cloves garlic, minced
1 zucchini, diced
1 cup green beans, trimmed and cut into 1/2-inch pieces
1 bell pepper, diced
1 can (15 oz) diced tomatoes
1 can (15 oz) cannellini beans, drained and rinsed
6 cups gluten-free vegetable broth
1 tsp dried oregano
1 tsp dried basil
1/2 cup gluten-free pasta (small shapes like macaroni or shells)
Salt and pepper to taste
Fresh parsley, chopped (for garnish)

Grated Parmesan cheese (ensure it's gluten-free, for serving)
Instructions:
Heat the olive oil in a large pot over medium heat. Add the onion, carrots, and celery, and sauté until softened.
Add the garlic, zucchini, green beans, and bell pepper. Cook for another 5 minutes.
Stir in the diced tomatoes, cannellini beans, vegetable broth, oregano, and basil. Bring to a boil.
Reduce heat to low and simmer for 20 minutes.
Add the gluten-free pasta and cook until al dente, about 10 minutes.
Season with salt and pepper. Serve hot, garnished with fresh parsley and grated Parmesan cheese.

Thai Coconut Soup
Ingredients:
1 tbsp coconut oil
1 small onion, thinly sliced
2 cloves garlic, minced
1 tbsp fresh ginger, grated
1 lemongrass stalk, pounded and cut into 2-inch pieces
1 red chili, sliced (optional for heat)
4 cups gluten-free chicken or vegetable broth
1 can (13.5 oz) coconut milk
1 tbsp fish sauce (ensure it's gluten-free)
1 tsp sugar
1 cup mushrooms, sliced
1 cup shrimp, peeled and deveined (optional)
Juice of 1 lime
Fresh cilantro leaves for garnish
Instructions:

Heat the coconut oil in a pot over medium heat. Add the onion, garlic, ginger, lemongrass, and chili (if using). Sauté until the onion is translucent.

Pour in the broth and bring to a simmer. Add the coconut milk, fish sauce, and sugar, stirring well.

Add the mushrooms and shrimp (if using). Cook until the shrimp are pink and cooked through.

Remove from heat and stir in the lime juice.

Serve hot, garnished with fresh cilantro leaves.

Beef Stew

Ingredients:

2 lbs beef chuck, cut into 1-inch cubes

1/4 cup gluten-free all-purpose flour

3 tbsp olive oil

1 large onion, chopped

3 cloves garlic, minced

3 carrots, peeled and sliced

2 celery stalks, sliced

1/4 cup tomato paste

4 cups gluten-free beef broth

1 cup red wine (ensure it's gluten-free)

2 bay leaves

1 tsp dried thyme

1 tsp smoked paprika

2 cups baby potatoes, halved

Salt and pepper to taste

Fresh parsley, chopped (for garnish)

Instructions:

Toss the beef cubes with the gluten-free flour to coat evenly.
Heat 2 tablespoons of olive oil in a large pot over medium-high heat.
Brown the beef on all sides. Remove the beef and set aside.
In the same pot, add the remaining olive oil, onion, garlic, carrots, and celery. Sauté until the vegetables are softened.
Stir in the tomato paste and cook for 1 minute.
Add the beef back to the pot along with the beef broth, red wine, bay leaves, thyme, and smoked paprika. Bring to a boil.
Reduce the heat to low, cover, and simmer for 1 hour.
Add the potatoes and continue to simmer until the beef and potatoes are tender, about 30 minutes.
Season with salt and pepper to taste. Serve hot, garnished with fresh parsley.

Lentil Soup
Ingredients:
2 tbsp olive oil
1 medium onion, diced
2 carrots, peeled and diced
2 stalks celery, diced
3 cloves garlic, minced
1 cup dried green lentils, rinsed
4 cups gluten-free vegetable broth
1 can (14.5 oz) diced tomatoes
1 tsp ground cumin
1/2 tsp ground coriander
1/2 tsp smoked paprika
Salt and pepper to taste
Fresh lemon juice (from 1 lemon)
Fresh cilantro, chopped (for garnish)

Instructions:

Heat the olive oil in a large pot over medium heat. Add the onion, carrots, and celery, and cook until the vegetables are softened.
Add the garlic and cook for another minute until fragrant.
Stir in the lentils, vegetable broth, diced tomatoes, cumin, coriander, and smoked paprika. Bring to a boil.
Reduce the heat to low and simmer, covered, until the lentils are tender, about 30 minutes.
Season with salt and pepper to taste. Add the fresh lemon juice.
Serve hot, garnished with fresh cilantro.

French Onion Soup

Ingredients:

4 large yellow onions, thinly sliced
2 tablespoons unsalted butter
1 tablespoon olive oil
1 teaspoon sugar
1 tablespoon all-purpose gluten-free flour
6 cups gluten-free beef broth
1/2 cup dry white wine (ensure it's gluten-free)
1 bay leaf
1/2 teaspoon dried thyme
Salt and freshly ground black pepper to taste
4 slices of gluten-free bread, toasted
1 cup grated Gruyère cheese (ensure it's gluten-free)

Instructions:

In a large pot, melt the butter with the olive oil over medium heat.
Add the onions and sugar, and cook, stirring occasionally, until the onions are caramelized to a deep golden brown, about 30 minutes.

Sprinkle the flour over the onions and cook, stirring, for a few minutes to form a roux.

Slowly add the beef broth, wine, bay leaf, and thyme, stirring constantly to prevent lumps.

Bring to a simmer, then reduce the heat to low and cook for 30 minutes. Season with salt and pepper.

Preheat the broiler. Ladle the soup into oven-safe bowls. Place a slice of toasted bread on top of each, and sprinkle generously with grated Gruyère cheese.

Broil until the cheese is bubbly and golden brown, about 3-5 minutes. Serve hot.

Vegetable Soup
Ingredients:
2 tablespoons olive oil
1 medium onion, diced
2 cloves garlic, minced
2 carrots, peeled and diced
2 stalks celery, diced
1 small zucchini, diced
1 cup green beans, trimmed and cut into 1-inch pieces
1 bell pepper, diced
1 can (14 oz) diced tomatoes, with juice
6 cups gluten-free vegetable broth
1 teaspoon dried basil
1 teaspoon dried oregano
1/2 cup gluten-free pasta (small shapes like macaroni or shells)
Salt and freshly ground black pepper to taste
Fresh parsley, chopped (for garnish)
Instructions:

Heat the olive oil in a large pot over medium heat. Add the onion and garlic, and sauté until the onion is translucent.
Add the carrots, celery, zucchini, green beans, and bell pepper.
Cook for about 5 minutes, until the vegetables start to soften.
Stir in the diced tomatoes with their juice, vegetable broth, basil, and oregano. Bring to a boil.
Reduce the heat to a simmer and cook for 20 minutes.
Add the gluten-free pasta and cook until al dente, about 10 minutes.
Season with salt and pepper to taste. Serve hot, garnished with fresh parsley.

Clam Chowder
Ingredients:
2 cans (6.5 oz each) chopped clams in juice
4 slices bacon, diced
1 large onion, chopped
2 cloves garlic, minced
3 medium potatoes, peeled and cubed
1 cup celery, diced
2 cups gluten-free chicken broth
1 cup heavy cream
1/4 cup gluten-free all-purpose flour
2 bay leaves
1 tsp dried thyme
Salt and pepper to taste
Fresh parsley, chopped (for garnish)
Instructions:
In a large pot, cook the bacon over medium heat until crisp. Remove bacon and set aside, leaving the drippings in the pot.
Add the onion and garlic to the pot and sauté until translucent.

Sprinkle the flour over the onions and garlic, stirring to create a roux. Gradually pour in the chicken broth, stirring constantly. Add the potatoes, celery, bay leaves, and thyme. Bring to a boil, then reduce heat and simmer until potatoes are tender.

Drain the clam juice from the cans into the pot and add the chopped clams during the last 5 minutes of cooking to prevent them from becoming tough.

Stir in the heavy cream and season with salt and pepper. Cook until heated through.

Serve hot, garnished with the cooked bacon and fresh parsley.

Pumpkin Soup

Ingredients:

1 medium pumpkin (about 3 lbs), peeled, seeded, and cubed

2 tbsp olive oil

1 large onion, diced

3 cloves garlic, minced

4 cups gluten-free vegetable broth

1 cup coconut milk

1 tsp ground cinnamon

1/2 tsp ground nutmeg

1/4 tsp ground ginger

Salt and pepper to taste

Roasted pumpkin seeds (for garnish)

Instructions:

Preheat your oven to 400°F (200°C). Toss the pumpkin cubes with olive oil and spread on a baking sheet. Roast for 30 minutes until tender and slightly caramelized.

In a large pot, heat a tablespoon of olive oil over medium heat. Add the onion and garlic, and cook until soft.

Add the roasted pumpkin to the pot along with the vegetable broth.
Bring to a simmer and cook for 10 minutes.
Use an immersion blender to purée the soup until smooth.
Stir in the coconut milk, cinnamon, nutmeg, and ginger. Season with salt and pepper to taste. Heat through.
Serve hot, garnished with roasted pumpkin seeds.

Spicy Black Bean Soup
Ingredients:
2 cups dried black beans, soaked overnight and drained
2 tablespoons olive oil
1 large onion, diced
3 cloves garlic, minced
1 red bell pepper, diced
1 green bell pepper, diced
1 jalapeño, seeded and minced
1 tablespoon ground cumin
1 teaspoon smoked paprika
1/2 teaspoon cayenne pepper (adjust to heat preference)
4 cups gluten-free vegetable broth
1 can (14 oz) diced tomatoes with green chilies
1 teaspoon dried oregano
Salt and pepper to taste
Fresh cilantro, chopped (for garnish)
Avocado slices (for garnish)
Lime wedges (for serving)
Instructions:
Heat the olive oil in a large pot over medium heat. Add the onion, garlic, bell peppers, and jalapeño. Cook until the vegetables are softened, about 5 minutes.

Stir in the cumin, smoked paprika, and cayenne pepper, and cook for another minute until fragrant.
Add the soaked black beans, vegetable broth, and diced tomatoes with green chilies. Bring to a boil.
Reduce the heat to low, cover, and simmer for about 1.5 to 2 hours, or until the beans are tender.
Use an immersion blender to puree part of the soup if a creamier texture is desired, or leave as is for a more rustic feel.
Season with oregano, salt, and pepper. Let the soup simmer for another 10 minutes.
Serve hot, garnished with fresh cilantro, avocado slices, and a squeeze of lime juice.

Unique Miso Soup
Ingredients:
4 cups gluten-free dashi stock
3 tablespoons gluten-free miso paste
1 block firm tofu, cut into 1/2-inch cubes
1/4 cup wakame seaweed, rehydrated
1/2 cup shiitake mushrooms, thinly sliced
2 green onions, thinly sliced
1 teaspoon grated ginger
Instructions:
In a pot, bring the dashi stock to a simmer over medium heat.
Place the miso paste in a small bowl, add a little hot stock, and whisk until smooth.
Add the miso mixture back into the pot with dashi, stirring gently to combine.
Add the tofu, wakame, and shiitake mushrooms to the pot and simmer for about 5 minutes.

Stir in the grated ginger and green onions, and simmer for another minute.
Serve hot, garnished with additional green onions if desired.

Unique Corn Chowder
Ingredients:
5 ears of fresh corn, kernels removed and cobs reserved
1 tablespoon olive oil
1 medium onion, diced
2 cloves garlic, minced
1 red bell pepper, diced
1 potato, peeled and diced
4 cups gluten-free vegetable broth
1 cup coconut milk
1/2 teaspoon smoked paprika
Salt and pepper to taste
Fresh chives, chopped (for garnish)
Instructions:
In a large pot, heat the olive oil over medium heat. Add the onion, garlic, and bell pepper, and sauté until softened.
Add the potato and corn kernels, cooking for another 5 minutes.
Pour in the vegetable broth and bring to a boil. Add the reserved corn cobs to the pot and simmer for 20 minutes.
Remove the cobs, then add the coconut milk and smoked paprika. Season with salt and pepper.
Use an immersion blender to blend about half of the soup directly in the pot until creamy but still chunky.
Serve hot, garnished with fresh chives.

Broccoli Salad with Sesame, Cumin & Garlic Ingredients:

Fresh broccoli florets
Red wine vinegar
Olive oil
Cumin seeds
Garlic, finely chopped
Sesame seeds
Instructions:
Lightly "pickle" the broccoli florets by tossing them in red wine
vinegar and let them sit for 10 minutes.
Toast the cumin seeds until fragrant and mix with finely chopped
garlic and sesame seeds.
Combine the olive oil with the cumin, garlic, and sesame mixture.
Toss the marinated broccoli in this dressing and let it sit to absorb
the flavors.

Quinoa Salad with Hoisin & Peanut Dressing Ingredients:
Cooked quinoa
Fresh vegetables (cucumber, red bell pepper, red onion)
Chickpeas
Fresh parsley
Hoisin sauce
Coconut milk
Peanut butter
Lime juice
Instructions:
Prepare the dressing by whisking together hoisin sauce, coconut
milk, peanut butter, and lime juice until smooth.
In a large bowl, combine the cooked quinoa with diced fresh
vegetables and chickpeas.
Chop the fresh parsley and add it to the bowl.

Drizzle the hoisin and peanut dressing over the salad and toss everything together until well mixed.

Greek Salad with Marinated Feta and Herbs Ingredients:
Ripe tomatoes, cut into wedges
Sliced cucumber
Thinly sliced red onion
Kalamata olives
Block of feta cheese
Olive oil
Red wine vinegar
Fresh dill, parsley, and mint, finely chopped
Lemon zest
Garlic, minced
Sea salt and freshly ground black pepper
Instructions:
In a bowl, whisk together olive oil, red wine vinegar, lemon zest, minced garlic, and herbs to create a marinade.
Place the block of feta in a shallow dish and pour the marinade over it. Let it marinate for at least 30 minutes.
Arrange the tomatoes, cucumber, red onion, and olives on a platter.
Take the marinated feta and crumble it over the salad.
Drizzle some of the marinade over the salad and season with salt and pepper to taste.

Cobb Salad with Citrus-Honey Vinaigrette
Ingredients:
Mixed greens (such as romaine, watercress, endive)
Cooked chicken breast, diced
Crispy bacon, crumbled

Hard-boiled eggs, sliced
Avocado, diced
Cherry tomatoes, halved
Blue cheese, crumbled
For the dressing:
Olive oil
Honey
Fresh orange juice
Fresh lemon juice
Dijon mustard
Salt and pepper
Instructions:
In a small bowl, whisk together olive oil, honey, orange juice, lemon juice, and Dijon mustard. Season with salt and pepper to taste.
On a large platter, arrange the mixed greens as a base.
Neatly arrange rows of chicken, bacon, eggs, avocado, tomatoes, and blue cheese over the greens.
Drizzle the citrus-honey vinaigrette over the salad just before serving.

Cool Beans Salad with a Mediterranean Twist Ingredients:
3 cups cooked basmati rice
1 can kidney beans, rinsed and drained
1 can black beans, rinsed and drained
1 1/2 cups frozen corn, thawed
4 green onions, sliced
1 small sweet red pepper, chopped
1/4 cup minced fresh parsley
1/2 cup feta cheese, crumbled
1/4 cup Kalamata olives, pitted and halved

For the dressing:
1/2 cup olive oil
1/4 cup lemon juice
1 tablespoon honey
1 garlic clove, minced
1 teaspoon salt
1 teaspoon ground cumin
1 teaspoon chili powder
1/4 teaspoon pepper
Instructions:
In a large bowl, whisk together the olive oil, lemon juice, honey, minced garlic, salt, cumin, chili powder, and pepper to create the dressing.
Add the cooked basmati rice, kidney beans, black beans, corn, green onions, sweet red pepper, parsley, feta cheese, and Kalamata olives to the bowl.
Toss everything together until well coated with the dressing.
Chill in the refrigerator for at least 30 minutes before serving to allow the flavors to meld.

Ribbon Salad with Orange Vinaigrette and Toasted Almonds
Ingredients:
1 medium zucchini
1 medium cucumber
1 medium carrot
3 medium oranges
3 cups fresh baby spinach
4 green onions, finely chopped
1/2 cup toasted almonds, sliced
1/2 teaspoon salt

1/2 teaspoon pepper
1/2 cup golden raisins (optional)
For the vinaigrette:
1/4 cup olive oil
4 teaspoons white wine vinegar
1 tablespoon finely chopped green onion
2 teaspoons honey
1/4 teaspoon salt
1/4 teaspoon pepper
Instructions:
Using a vegetable peeler, shave the zucchini, cucumber, and carrot lengthwise into very thin strips.
Finely grate enough zest from the oranges to measure 2 tablespoons. Cut one orange crosswise in half; squeeze juice from the orange to measure 1/2 cup. Reserve zest and juice for the vinaigrette.
Cut a thin slice from the top and bottom of the remaining oranges; stand oranges upright on a cutting board. With a knife, cut off the peel and outer membrane from the oranges. Cut along the membrane of each segment to remove the fruit.
In a large bowl, combine the spinach, orange sections, green onions, toasted almonds, salt, pepper, and, if desired, raisins.
Add the vegetable ribbons and gently toss to combine.
In a small bowl, whisk together the vinaigrette ingredients, including the reserved orange zest and juice.
Drizzle half of the vinaigrette over the salad and toss to coat. Serve with the remaining vinaigrette.

Roasted Beet Salad with Orange and Pistachios Ingredients:
4 medium beets, roasted and sliced

2 oranges, peeled and segmented
1/2 cup of shelled pistachios, toasted
1/4 cup of crumbled goat cheese
Mixed greens (such as arugula or spinach)
For the dressing:
3 tablespoons extra virgin olive oil
1 tablespoon balsamic vinegar
1 tablespoon orange juice
1 teaspoon honey
Salt and pepper to taste
Instructions:
Preheat your oven to 400°F (200°C). Wrap the beets in foil and roast until tender, about 45 minutes. Let cool, peel, and slice[1].
In a dry skillet, toast the pistachios over medium heat until fragrant. Set aside to cool.
In a small bowl, whisk together the olive oil, balsamic vinegar, orange juice, and honey. Season with salt and pepper.
Arrange the mixed greens on a platter. Top with the roasted beet slices and orange segments.
Sprinkle the toasted pistachios and crumbled goat cheese over the salad.
Drizzle the dressing over the salad just before serving.

Chipotle Lime Avocado Salad
Ingredients:
2 ripe avocados, diced
1 cup cherry tomatoes, halved
1/2 red onion, finely chopped
1 can black beans, rinsed and drained
1 cup corn kernels, fresh or thawed from frozen

1/4 cup fresh cilantro, chopped
For the dressing:
2 tablespoons lime juice
1 tablespoon chipotle in adobo sauce, finely chopped
1/4 cup olive oil
1 teaspoon honey
Salt and pepper to taste
Instructions:
In a large bowl, combine the diced avocados, cherry tomatoes, red onion, black beans, and corn.
In a small bowl, whisk together the lime juice, chipotle in adobo sauce, olive oil, and honey. Season with salt and pepper.
Pour the dressing over the salad ingredients and gently toss to combine.
Garnish with chopped cilantro just before serving.

Green Salad with Shrimp and Pomegranate Wine Vinaigrette
Ingredients:
6 cups mixed greens (like arugula, spinach, and romaine)
20 large shrimp, peeled and deveined
1 avocado, sliced
1/2 cup pomegranate seeds
1/4 cup toasted pine nuts
For the vinaigrette:
1/4 cup red wine vinegar
1/4 cup pomegranate juice
1/2 cup extra virgin olive oil
1 tablespoon honey
1 teaspoon Dijon mustard
Salt and pepper to taste

Instructions:
Season the shrimp with salt and pepper, and sauté in a pan over medium heat until pink and cooked through. Set aside to cool.
In a bowl, whisk together the red wine vinegar, pomegranate juice, olive oil, honey, and Dijon mustard. Season with salt and pepper.
In a large salad bowl, toss the mixed greens with the vinaigrette.
Top the salad with the cooled shrimp, avocado slices, pomegranate seeds, and toasted pine nuts.
Serve immediately and enjoy the burst of flavors!

Lemon Rice Salad with Fresh Herbs and Almonds
 Ingredients:
3 cups cooked jasmine rice, cooled
1/4 cup slivered almonds, toasted
1/4 cup fresh parsley, chopped
1/4 cup fresh mint, chopped
1/4 cup fresh dill, chopped
Zest and juice of 2 lemons
1/4 cup extra virgin olive oil
Salt and pepper to taste
Instructions:
In a large mixing bowl, combine the cooled jasmine rice with the toasted slivered almonds and fresh herbs.
In a small bowl, whisk together the lemon zest, lemon juice, and olive oil. Season with salt and pepper.
Pour the lemon dressing over the rice mixture and toss until everything is well coated.
Adjust the seasoning if necessary and chill in the refrigerator for at least 30 minutes before serving.

Enjoy this refreshing and zesty salad as a side dish or a light main course!

Bacon Pear Salad with Honey-Thyme Parmesan Dressing
Ingredients:
Mixed greens
2 ripe pears, sliced
4 strips of bacon, cooked and crumbled
1/4 cup toasted walnuts
1/4 cup crumbled blue cheese
For the dressing:
1/4 cup grated Parmesan cheese
1/4 cup olive oil
2 tablespoons honey
1 tablespoon white wine vinegar
1 teaspoon fresh thyme leaves
Salt and pepper to taste
Instructions:
In a large salad bowl, combine mixed greens, sliced pears, crumbled bacon, toasted walnuts, and blue cheese.
In a small bowl, whisk together the Parmesan cheese, olive oil, honey, white wine vinegar, and thyme leaves until well blended. Season with salt and pepper.
Drizzle the dressing over the salad and toss gently to coat. Serve immediately.

Cherry Tomato Salad with Balsamic Reduction Ingredients:
4 cups cherry tomatoes, halved
1/4 cup fresh basil leaves, torn

1/4 cup red onion, thinly sliced
1/4 cup feta cheese, crumbled
For the balsamic reduction:
1/2 cup balsamic vinegar
1 tablespoon brown sugar
Instructions:
In a small saucepan, combine balsamic vinegar and brown sugar. Simmer over medium heat until reduced by half and thickened, about 10 minutes. Allow to cool.
In a salad bowl, combine cherry tomatoes, basil leaves, red onion, and feta cheese.
Drizzle the cooled balsamic reduction over the salad just before serving.

Green Salad with Creamy Dill Dressing
Ingredients:
4 cups mixed salad greens (like baby spinach, arugula, and romaine)
1/2 cup cherry tomatoes, halved
1/4 cup cucumber, thinly sliced
1/4 cup red onion, thinly sliced
1/4 cup radishes, thinly sliced
2 tablespoons fresh dill, chopped
For the dressing:
1/4 cup Greek yogurt
2 tablespoons mayonnaise
1 tablespoon fresh lemon juice
1 teaspoon Dijon mustard
1 garlic clove, minced
Salt and pepper to taste
Instructions:

In a large salad bowl, combine the mixed greens, cherry tomatoes, cucumber, red onion, and radishes.

In a small bowl, whisk together the Greek yogurt, mayonnaise, lemon juice, Dijon mustard, and minced garlic until smooth. Stir in the chopped dill, and season with salt and pepper.

Drizzle the creamy dill dressing over the salad just before serving and toss to coat evenly.

Exotic Fresh Fruit Bowl with Minted Honey Drizzle

Ingredients:

1 cup pineapple, cubed

1 mango, peeled and cubed

1/2 cup kiwi, sliced

1/2 cup papaya, cubed

1/2 cup strawberries, halved

1/4 cup blueberries

Fresh mint leaves for garnish

For the drizzle:

2 tablespoons honey

1 tablespoon fresh lime juice

1 tablespoon water

1 teaspoon fresh mint, finely chopped

Instructions:

In a large serving bowl, combine the pineapple, mango, kiwi, papaya, strawberries, and blueberries.

In a small bowl, whisk together the honey, lime juice, water, and chopped mint until well combined.

Drizzle the minted honey over the fruit just before serving.

Garnish with fresh mint leaves for an extra touch of freshness.

Herby Pea Salad with Citrus-Mint Dressing

Ingredients:

3 cups fresh or frozen peas, blanched

1/4 cup fresh mint leaves, finely chopped

1/4 cup fresh basil leaves, finely chopped

1/4 cup fresh parsley, finely chopped

1/4 cup feta cheese, crumbled

1/4 cup toasted pine nuts

For the dressing:

3 tablespoons extra virgin olive oil

2 tablespoons fresh lemon juice

1 tablespoon fresh orange juice

1 teaspoon honey

Salt and pepper to taste

Instructions:

If using frozen peas, blanch them in boiling water for 1 minute, then plunge into ice water to stop the cooking process. Drain well.

In a large bowl, combine the blanched peas, chopped mint, basil, parsley, crumbled feta, and toasted pine nuts.

In a small bowl, whisk together the olive oil, lemon juice, orange juice, and honey. Season with salt and pepper to taste.

Pour the citrus-mint dressing over the pea mixture and toss gently to combine.

Chill in the refrigerator for about 30 minutes before serving to allow the flavors to meld.

Snacks and Appetizers

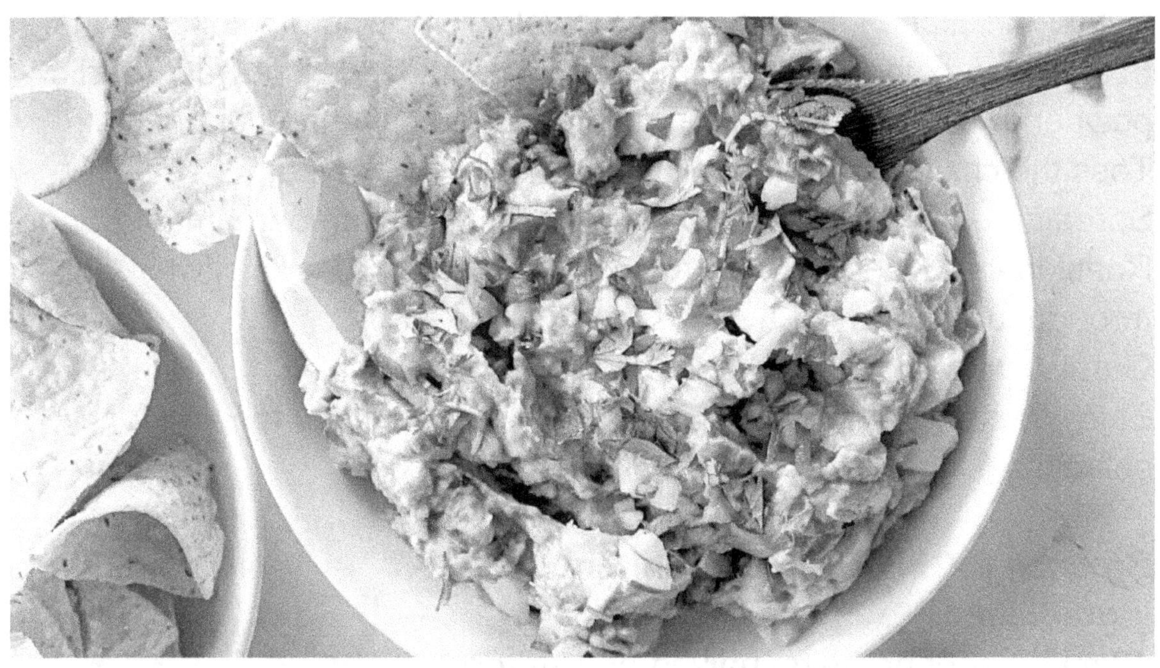

Chili Lime Roasted Chickpeas
Ingredients:
1 can (15 oz) chickpeas, drained and rinsed
1 tbsp olive oil
Zest of 1 lime
2 tbsp lime juice
1 tsp chili powder
1/2 tsp garlic powder
1/2 tsp onion powder
1/4 tsp cumin
1/4 tsp sea salt
1/8 tsp cayenne pepper (optional for extra heat)

Fresh cilantro for garnish
Instructions:
Preheat your oven to 400°F (200°C).
Pat the chickpeas dry with paper towels, removing any loose skins.
In a bowl, mix the olive oil, lime zest, lime juice, chili powder, garlic powder, onion powder, cumin, sea salt, and cayenne pepper.
Toss the chickpeas in the mixture until evenly coated.
Spread the chickpeas on a baking sheet lined with parchment paper.
Roast in the oven for 25-30 minutes, shaking the pan halfway through, until crispy.
Garnish with chopped cilantro before serving.
Enjoy these as a tangy, spicy snack or as a crunchy topping for salads!

Broccoli & Chive Stuffed Mini Peppers
Ingredients:
12 mini sweet peppers, halved and seeded
1 cup broccoli florets, finely chopped
4 oz cream cheese, softened
1/4 cup chives, finely chopped
1/2 cup shredded mozzarella cheese
1/4 tsp garlic powder
Salt and pepper to taste
Olive oil for drizzling
Instructions:
Preheat your oven to 375°F (190°C).
Steam the broccoli florets until just tender, then chop finely.
In a mixing bowl, combine the cream cheese, chives, garlic powder, salt, and pepper.
Fold in the steamed broccoli until the mixture is well combined.

Stuff each pepper half with the broccoli mixture and place on a baking tray.

Top each with a sprinkle of mozzarella cheese.

Drizzle a little olive oil over the peppers.

Bake for 10-12 minutes or until the peppers are tender and the cheese is bubbly and golden.

Serve warm as a delightful appetizer.

Cheese Crisp

Ingredients:

4 medium flour tortillas (the thinner, the better)

4 tsp unsalted butter, melted

2 cups grated cheese (a mix of cheddar and Oaxaca cheese works well)

Optional toppings: roasted green chiles, diced tomatoes, sliced olives

Instructions:

Preheat your oven to 325°F (163°C).

Brush both sides of the tortillas with melted butter.

Place the tortillas on a wire rack set over a baking sheet.

Bake for 20-25 minutes, turning halfway through, until they start to crisp.

Remove from the oven and sprinkle the grated cheese (and optional toppings) over the tortillas.

Increase the oven temperature to 450°F (232°C).

Return the tortillas to the oven for about 5 minutes, until the cheese bubbles and the edges are golden brown.

Enjoy this simple yet delicious Southwest favorite!

Ham Balls with Brown Sugar Glaze

Ingredients:
2 lbs ham loaf mix (or a mix of ground ham and ground pork)
2 eggs, slightly beaten
1/2 cup milk
1 cup soft bread crumbs
For the Glaze:
3/4 cup brown sugar
1 tbsp dry mustard
3/4 cup cider vinegar
3/4 cup hot water
Instructions:
Preheat your oven to 350°F (177°C).
In a medium bowl, soak the bread crumbs in milk for about 5 minutes.
Stir in the eggs, then add the meat mix and combine well.
Shape the mixture into balls and place them in a greased 9x13 inch pan.
In a separate bowl, mix together the brown sugar, dry mustard, cider vinegar, and hot water for the glaze.
Pour the glaze over the ham balls.
Bake for 2 hours, basting occasionally with the sauce

Unique Baba Ganoush
Ingredients:
2 medium-sized eggplants
3 tbsp tahini
2 garlic cloves, minced
2 tbsp fresh lemon juice

1/4 cup olive oil, plus more for garnish
Salt to taste
1/2 tsp smoked paprika
1/4 tsp ground cumin
1 tbsp chopped parsley
1 tbsp pomegranate seeds (optional)
Instructions:
Preheat your oven to 400°F (200°C).
Prick the eggplants with a fork and place them on a baking sheet.
Roast in the oven for 35-40 minutes until the skin is charred and the inside is soft.
Remove from oven and let cool. Peel off the skin and discard.
In a bowl, mash the eggplant with a fork or blend in a food processor for a smoother texture.
Add tahini, minced garlic, lemon juice, and olive oil. Mix until well combined.
Season with salt, smoked paprika, and ground cumin.
Transfer to a serving dish, drizzle with olive oil, and garnish with chopped parsley and pomegranate seeds for a pop of color and sweetness.
Serve with gluten-free pita bread or vegetable sticks.

Unique Coconut Shrimp
Ingredients:
1 lb large shrimp, peeled and deveined
1/2 cup cornstarch
1/2 tsp salt
1/2 tsp cayenne pepper
2 large eggs, beaten
1 cup shredded unsweetened coconut

1 cup panko breadcrumbs (gluten-free if necessary)
Vegetable oil for frying
For the Dipping Sauce:
1/2 cup orange marmalade
1 tbsp rice vinegar
1 tbsp soy sauce (gluten-free if necessary)
1/2 tsp crushed red pepper flakes
Instructions:
In a shallow bowl, combine cornstarch, salt, and cayenne pepper.
Place beaten eggs in another bowl, and mix shredded coconut with
panko breadcrumbs in a third bowl.
Dredge each shrimp in the cornstarch mixture, dip into the eggs,
then coat with the coconut-panko mixture.
Heat vegetable oil in a large frying pan over medium-high heat.
Fry the shrimp in batches until golden brown, about 2-3 minutes per
side.
For the dipping sauce, combine orange marmalade, rice vinegar, soy
sauce, and red pepper flakes in a small bowl.
Serve the shrimp hot with the dipping sauce on the side.

Air Fryer Sweet Potato Chips
Ingredients:
2 large sweet potatoes, peeled
1 tbsp olive oil
1 tsp smoked paprika
1/2 tsp garlic powder
1/2 tsp onion powder
Salt to taste
Freshly ground black pepper to taste
Instructions:

Thinly slice the sweet potatoes using a mandoline slicer for uniform thickness.

In a bowl, toss the sweet potato slices with olive oil, smoked paprika, garlic powder, onion powder, salt, and pepper until evenly coated.

Preheat the air fryer to 360°F (182°C).

Arrange the sweet potato slices in a single layer in the air fryer basket, ensuring they don't overlap for even cooking.

Air fry for 10-12 minutes, flipping halfway through, until the chips are crispy and golden brown.

Let them cool for a few minutes to crisp up further before serving.

Enjoy these smoky and savory sweet potato chips as a healthy snack!

Habanero and Mango Guacamole

Ingredients:

3 ripe avocados, halved, pitted, and scooped out

1 ripe mango, diced

1 habanero pepper, finely chopped (remove seeds for less heat)

Juice of 1 lime

1/4 cup red onion, finely diced

1/4 cup fresh cilantro, chopped

Salt to taste

Instructions:

In a large bowl, mash the avocados to your desired consistency.

Add the diced mango, habanero pepper, lime juice, red onion, and cilantro to the mashed avocados.

Gently fold the ingredients together until well combined.

Season with salt to taste and give it one final mix.

Let the guacamole sit for about 10 minutes to allow the flavors to meld together.
Serve with tortilla chips or fresh veggies for dipping.

Red Lentil Hummus with Crispy Brussels Sprouts
Ingredients:
1 cup red lentils
2 cups water
2 tbsp tahini
2 garlic cloves, minced
4 tbsp olive oil, divided
Juice of 1 lemon
Salt and pepper to taste
1/2 tsp cumin
1/2 tsp smoked paprika
2 cups Brussels sprouts, trimmed and halved
1 tbsp balsamic vinegar
Instructions:
Rinse the red lentils and bring them to a boil in 2 cups of water. Reduce heat and simmer until tender, about 15 minutes. Drain and let cool.
In a food processor, blend the cooked lentils, tahini, garlic, 2 tbsp olive oil, lemon juice, cumin, smoked paprika, salt, and pepper until smooth.
Preheat your oven to 400°F (200°C).
Toss the Brussels sprouts with the remaining 2 tbsp olive oil, balsamic vinegar, salt, and pepper.
Spread the Brussels sprouts on a baking sheet and roast until crispy, about 20-25 minutes.

Serve the hummus topped with the crispy Brussels sprouts and a drizzle of olive oil.

Enjoy this hearty and flavorful twist on traditional hummus!

Bacon and Fontina Stuffed Mushrooms

Ingredients:

24 large fresh mushrooms, stems removed

8 slices bacon, cooked and crumbled

1 cup fontina cheese, shredded

4 oz cream cheese, softened

1/4 cup green onions, chopped

1/4 cup sun-dried tomatoes, chopped

3 tbsp fresh parsley, minced

1 tbsp olive oil

Salt and pepper to taste

Instructions:

Preheat your oven to 425°F (220°C).

In a bowl, mix together the crumbled bacon, fontina cheese, cream cheese, green onions, sun-dried tomatoes, parsley, salt, and pepper until well combined.

Stuff each mushroom cap with the mixture and arrange them on a greased baking sheet.

Drizzle the tops with olive oil.

Bake for 9-11 minutes or until the mushrooms are tender and the tops are golden brown.

Herb Roasted Olives & Tomatoes

Ingredients:

2 cups mixed olives (Kalamata, green, and black)

1 pint cherry tomatoes

4 cloves garlic, minced
1/4 cup extra virgin olive oil
1 tbsp fresh rosemary, chopped
1 tbsp fresh thyme, chopped
Zest of 1 lemon
Salt and pepper to taste
Instructions:
Preheat your oven to 400°F (200°C).
In a mixing bowl, combine olives, cherry tomatoes, and minced garlic.
Drizzle with olive oil and add the chopped rosemary, thyme, and lemon zest. Season with salt and pepper.
Toss everything together until well coated.
Spread the mixture on a baking sheet in a single layer.
Roast for 20-25 minutes, stirring occasionally, until the tomatoes are blistered and the olives are slightly caramelized.
Serve warm with crusty gluten-free bread or as a complement to a cheese platter.
Enjoy this Mediterranean-inspired dish that's bursting with flavor!

Orange Chicken Meatballs
Ingredients:
1 lb ground chicken
1/4 cup almond flour
1 large egg
2 tbsp orange zest
1/4 cup fresh orange juice
2 cloves garlic, minced
1 tbsp fresh ginger, grated
2 tbsp soy sauce (gluten-free if necessary)

1 tbsp honey
1 tsp sesame oil
Salt and pepper to taste
For the Glaze:
1/2 cup orange marmalade
2 tbsp soy sauce (gluten-free if necessary)
1 tbsp rice vinegar
1 tbsp honey
1/2 tsp garlic powder
1/2 tsp ginger powder
1 tbsp water
1 tsp cornstarch
Instructions:
Preheat your oven to 375°F (190°C).
In a bowl, combine ground chicken, almond flour, egg, orange zest, orange juice, minced garlic, grated ginger, soy sauce, honey, sesame oil, salt, and pepper. Mix until well combined.
Form the mixture into 1-inch meatballs and place on a baking sheet lined with parchment paper.
Bake for 20-25 minutes, or until the meatballs are cooked through.
While the meatballs are baking, prepare the glaze by combining all the glaze ingredients in a saucepan over medium heat.
Stir until the mixture thickens and becomes glossy.
Once the meatballs are done, toss them in the glaze until well coated.
Serve the meatballs over a bed of steamed rice or with toothpicks as an appetizer.

Sausage & Sage Stuffed Mushrooms
Ingredients:

24 large cremini mushrooms, stems removed
1/2 lb ground sausage
1/4 cup fresh sage, finely chopped
1/2 cup grated Parmesan cheese
1/4 cup breadcrumbs (gluten-free if needed)
1/4 cup cream cheese, softened
2 cloves garlic, minced
1 small onion, finely diced
2 tbsp olive oil
Salt and pepper to taste

Instructions:

Preheat your oven to 375°F (190°C).

In a skillet, heat 1 tbsp olive oil over medium heat. Add the sausage, onion, and garlic, and cook until the sausage is browned and the onions are translucent.

Stir in the sage, breadcrumbs, and half of the Parmesan cheese until well combined. Remove from heat and mix in the cream cheese.

Brush the mushroom caps with the remaining olive oil and season with salt and pepper.

Spoon the sausage mixture into the mushroom caps and place them on a baking sheet.

Sprinkle the remaining Parmesan cheese over the stuffed mushrooms.

Bake for 20 minutes or until the mushrooms are tender and the tops are golden brown.

Enjoy these savory stuffed mushrooms as a delightful appetizer or side dish!

Honey Lemon Pepper Chicken Wings
Ingredients:

2 lbs chicken wings, tips removed, drumettes and flats separated
1 tbsp baking powder
1 tsp salt
1/2 tsp black pepper
1/2 tsp garlic powder
Zest and juice of 2 lemons
1/4 cup honey
1 tbsp lemon pepper seasoning
1/4 cup butter, melted

Instructions:

Preheat your oven to 425°F (220°C). Line a baking sheet with foil and place a wire rack on top.

Pat the chicken wings dry with paper towels. In a large bowl, mix the baking powder, salt, pepper, and garlic powder.

Toss the wings in the seasoning mixture until they are evenly coated. Arrange the wings on the wire rack and bake for 45-50 minutes, flipping halfway through, until crispy and golden.

While the wings are baking, whisk together the lemon zest, lemon juice, honey, lemon pepper seasoning, and melted butter in a bowl.

Once the wings are done, toss them in the honey lemon pepper sauce until evenly coated.

Serve the wings immediately, garnished with extra lemon zest if desired.

Crockpot Buffalo Turkey Meatballs
Ingredients:
1 lb ground turkey
1/4 cup almond flour
1 large egg

1/4 cup hot sauce (like Frank's Red Hot)
1/4 cup unsalted butter, melted
1/2 tsp garlic powder
1/2 tsp onion powder
Salt and pepper to taste
1/4 cup blue cheese crumbles
Fresh parsley for garnish

Instructions:

In a large bowl, combine the ground turkey, almond flour, egg, garlic powder, onion powder, salt, and pepper. Mix until just combined.
Form the mixture into small, bite-sized meatballs.
Place the meatballs in the crockpot.
In a separate bowl, whisk together the hot sauce and melted butter.
Pour the buffalo sauce over the meatballs in the crockpot.
Cook on low for 4-6 hours or on high for 2-3 hours, until the meatballs are cooked through.
Sprinkle blue cheese crumbles over the meatballs and garnish with chopped parsley before serving.
Enjoy these spicy and tangy meatballs as an appetizer or main dish!

Zucchini Sliders

Ingredients:

2 large zucchinis, cut into 1/2 inch thick rounds
1 lb lean ground beef
Salt and pepper to taste
1 tsp Worcestershire sauce
1/2 cup cheddar cheese, sliced into small squares
1 tbsp olive oil
Optional toppings: lettuce, tomato, onion, pickles

Instructions:

Season the ground beef with salt, pepper, and Worcestershire sauce. Form into small patties that will fit your zucchini rounds. Heat olive oil in a skillet over medium-high heat. Cook the beef patties for about 3-4 minutes on each side or until desired doneness. While the patties are cooking, grill or pan-fry the zucchini rounds until tender and slightly charred, about 2 minutes per side.

Assemble the sliders by placing a beef patty on one zucchini round, add a slice of cheese, and any other toppings you like, then top with another zucchini round.

Gluten-Free Meatballs
Ingredients:
1 lb ground beef (preferably 90% lean)
1 lb ground pork or Italian sausage
4 slices gluten-free white bread, crusts removed and torn into pieces
1/2 cup milk (or a dairy-free alternative)
1/4 cup freshly grated Parmesan cheese
1/4 cup fresh parsley, finely chopped
2 large eggs
2 cloves garlic, minced
1 small onion, grated (include the juices)
1 tsp salt
1/2 tsp black pepper
2 tbsp olive oil (for frying)
Instructions:
Soak the gluten-free bread pieces in milk until soft.
In a large bowl, combine the ground beef and pork.
Squeeze the excess milk from the bread and add to the meat.
Mix in Parmesan, parsley, eggs, garlic, onion, salt, and pepper.
Form into 1-inch meatballs.

Heat olive oil in a skillet over medium heat and brown the meatballs on all sides.

Transfer to a baking sheet and bake at 375°F (190°C) for 20-25 minutes, or until cooked through.

Serve with your favorite gluten-free pasta and sauce for a classic Italian meal.

Del Real Carnitas

Ingredients:

2 lbs pork shoulder, cut into 2-inch chunks

1 orange, juice and zest

1 lime, juice and zest

4 cloves garlic, minced

1 onion, chopped

1 tsp ground cumin

1 tsp dried oregano

Salt and pepper to taste

2 tbsp vegetable oil

1/4 cup chicken broth

Instructions:

Season the pork chunks with salt, pepper, cumin, and oregano.

In a large skillet, heat the vegetable oil over medium-high heat.

Brown the pork chunks on all sides.

Transfer the pork to a crockpot.

Add the garlic, onion, orange juice and zest, lime juice and zest, and chicken broth.

Cook on low for 8 hours or until the pork is tender and shreds easily.

Shred the pork with two forks and, if desired, crisp up in a skillet before serving.

Applegate Chicken & Apple Sausage with Caramelized Onion and Apple Relish

Ingredients:

1 package Applegate Chicken & Apple Sausages

2 tbsp olive oil

2 large onions, thinly sliced

2 apples, cored and sliced

2 tbsp balsamic vinegar

1 tbsp brown sugar

Salt and pepper to taste

Fresh thyme leaves for garnish

Instructions:

Heat 1 tbsp of olive oil in a skillet over medium heat.

Add the sausages and cook until browned on all sides and heated through. Remove from the skillet and set aside.

In the same skillet, add the remaining olive oil, onions, and apples. Cook until the onions are soft and golden.

Stir in balsamic vinegar and brown sugar, and continue to cook until the mixture is thickened and caramelized.

Season with salt and pepper to taste.

Serve the sausages topped with the caramelized onion and apple relish and garnished with fresh thyme leaves.

Enjoy this sweet and savory dish that's perfect for a cozy dinner!

Stubb's BBQ Sauce Glazed Wings with a Honey Mustard Twist

Ingredients:

2 lbs chicken wings, tips removed, drumettes and flats separated

Salt and pepper to taste

1 cup Stubb's BBQ Sauce

2 tbsp honey
2 tbsp Dijon mustard
1 tbsp apple cider vinegar
1/4 tsp garlic powder
1/4 tsp onion powder
1 tbsp butter, melted

Instructions:

Preheat your oven to 400°F (200°C). Line a baking sheet with foil and place a wire rack on top.

Season the chicken wings with salt and pepper, and arrange them on the wire rack.

Bake for 45-50 minutes, or until the wings are crispy and fully cooked.

While the wings are baking, combine Stubb's BBQ Sauce, honey, Dijon mustard, apple cider vinegar, garlic powder, and onion powder in a saucepan over medium heat.

Bring the sauce to a simmer and cook until slightly thickened, about 5-7 minutes.

Remove from heat and stir in the melted butter.

Once the wings are done, toss them in the sauce until they are well coated.

Serve the wings hot, garnished with your choice of herbs or dipping sauces.

Caprese Skewers with Balsamic Glaze
Ingredients:
16 cherry tomatoes
16 fresh mozzarella balls (Ciliegine)
16 fresh basil leaves

2 tbsp extra virgin olive oil
Salt and freshly ground black pepper to taste
1/4 cup balsamic vinegar
1 tsp honey
Instructions:
In a small saucepan, combine balsamic vinegar and honey. Simmer over low heat until the mixture reduces by half and becomes syrupy, about 10 minutes. Allow to cool.
Assemble the skewers by threading a cherry tomato, a basil leaf folded in half, and a mozzarella ball onto each skewer. Repeat the process until all ingredients are used.
Arrange the skewers on a platter. Drizzle with olive oil and season with salt and pepper.
Just before serving, drizzle the balsamic glaze over the skewers.
Enjoy these skewers as a refreshing and elegant appetizer!

Gluten-Free Bruschetta
Ingredients:
1 gluten-free baguette, sliced into 1/2-inch rounds
4 tbsp olive oil
2 cups ripe tomatoes, diced
1/4 cup red onion, finely chopped
2 cloves garlic, minced
1/4 cup fresh basil, chopped
2 tbsp balsamic vinegar
Salt and pepper to taste
Instructions:
Preheat your oven to 350°F (175°C).
Brush both sides of each baguette slice with olive oil and place them on a baking sheet.

Toast in the oven for 10-15 minutes, or until golden and crisp.
In a mixing bowl, combine diced tomatoes, red onion, garlic, basil, and balsamic vinegar. Season with salt and pepper.
Spoon the tomato mixture generously onto each toasted baguette slice.

Quinoa Salad Stuffed Avocados
Ingredients:
2 ripe avocados, halved and pitted
1 cup cooked quinoa
1/2 cup cherry tomatoes, halved
1/4 cup red onion, finely chopped
1/4 cup cucumber, diced
1/4 cup feta cheese, crumbled
2 tbsp fresh cilantro, chopped
Juice of 1 lime
Salt and pepper to taste
Drizzle of extra virgin olive oil
Instructions:
Scoop out a little of the avocado flesh to create a larger cavity for the filling.
In a bowl, mix together the cooked quinoa, cherry tomatoes, red onion, cucumber, feta cheese, and cilantro.
Squeeze lime juice over the mixture, add salt and pepper to taste, and toss gently.
Fill each avocado half with the quinoa salad mixture.
Drizzle with olive oil just before serving.

Enjoy this refreshing and nutritious dish as a light lunch or a healthy appetizer!

Gluten-Free Pita Chips with Hummus
Ingredients for Pita Chips:
4 gluten-free pita breads
1/4 cup olive oil
1 tsp garlic powder
1 tsp dried oregano
Salt to taste
Ingredients for Hummus:
1 can (15 oz) chickpeas, drained and rinsed
2 tbsp tahini
2 cloves garlic
Juice of 1 lemon
2 tbsp olive oil
Salt and pepper to taste
Paprika for garnish
Instructions:
Preheat your oven to 375°F (190°C).
Cut the pita bread into triangles and arrange them on a baking sheet.
Mix olive oil with garlic powder, dried oregano, and salt.
Brush the mixture over the pita triangles.
Bake for 10-15 minutes until golden and crispy.
For the hummus, blend chickpeas, tahini, garlic, lemon juice, and olive oil in a food processor until smooth.
Season with salt and pepper to taste.
Serve the pita chips with hummus, sprinkled with paprika.

Tito's Vodka Infused Watermelon
Ingredients:
1 medium seedless watermelon
1 bottle Tito's Handmade Vodka
Fresh mint leaves for garnish
Instructions:
Cut a circular hole at the top of the watermelon, deep enough to reach the center.
Using a spoon or melon baller, remove some watermelon flesh to create a well.
Insert the open bottle of Tito's Vodka into the hole.
Let the bottle sit for 4-5 days in a cool, dark place, allowing the vodka to infuse into the watermelon.
Once infused, remove the bottle and refrigerate the watermelon until chilled.
Slice the watermelon and serve with fresh mint leaves as garnish.
Enjoy this refreshing and spirited summer treat responsibly!

Toma Bloody Mary Mix Veggie Dip
Ingredients:
1 cup Toma Bloody Mary Mix
1 cup sour cream or Greek yogurt
1/2 cup cream cheese, softened
1 tbsp Worcestershire sauce
1 tsp hot sauce (adjust to taste)
1/2 tsp celery salt
1/2 tsp smoked paprika
Fresh vegetables for dipping (carrots, celery, bell peppers)
Instructions:

In a mixing bowl, combine the Toma Bloody Mary Mix, sour cream or Greek yogurt, and cream cheese. Mix until smooth.
Stir in Worcestershire sauce, hot sauce, celery salt, and smoked paprika.
Cover and refrigerate for at least 1 hour to allow the flavors to meld.
Serve chilled with an assortment of fresh vegetables for dipping.

Riega Organic Taco Seasoned Popcorn
Ingredients:
1/2 cup popcorn kernels
2 tbsp coconut oil (or vegetable oil)
2 tbsp Riega Organic Taco Seasoning
1/4 cup nutritional yeast (for a cheesy flavor)
1 tsp lime zest
Salt to taste
Instructions:
Heat the coconut oil in a large pot over medium heat.
Once the oil is hot, add the popcorn kernels and cover with a lid.
Shake the pot occasionally as the kernels pop.
Once the popping slows down to more than 2 seconds between pops, remove from heat.
Sprinkle the Riega Organic Taco Seasoning, nutritional yeast, and lime zest over the popped corn.
Place the lid back on and shake the pot vigorously to evenly coat the popcorn.
Taste and add salt if needed.
Serve immediately and enjoy a zesty, savory snack

Lea & Perrins Worcestershire Sauce Marinated Steak
Ingredients:
4 steaks (your choice of cut)
1/2 cup Lea & Perrins Worcestershire Sauce
2 tbsp olive oil
2 cloves garlic, minced
1 tsp black pepper
1 tsp onion powder
1/2 tsp smoked paprika
1/2 tsp dried thyme
Instructions:
In a bowl, whisk together the Worcestershire sauce, olive oil, garlic, black pepper, onion powder, smoked paprika, and dried thyme.
Place the steaks in a large resealable plastic bag or shallow dish.
Pour the marinade over the steaks, ensuring they are well coated.
.Seal the bag or cover the dish and refrigerate for at least 2 hours, or overnight for deeper flavor.
Preheat your grill or skillet over medium-high heat.
Remove the steaks from the marinade and grill to your preferred level of doneness.
Let the steaks rest for a few minutes before serving to allow the juices to redistribute.

Meatless Mains

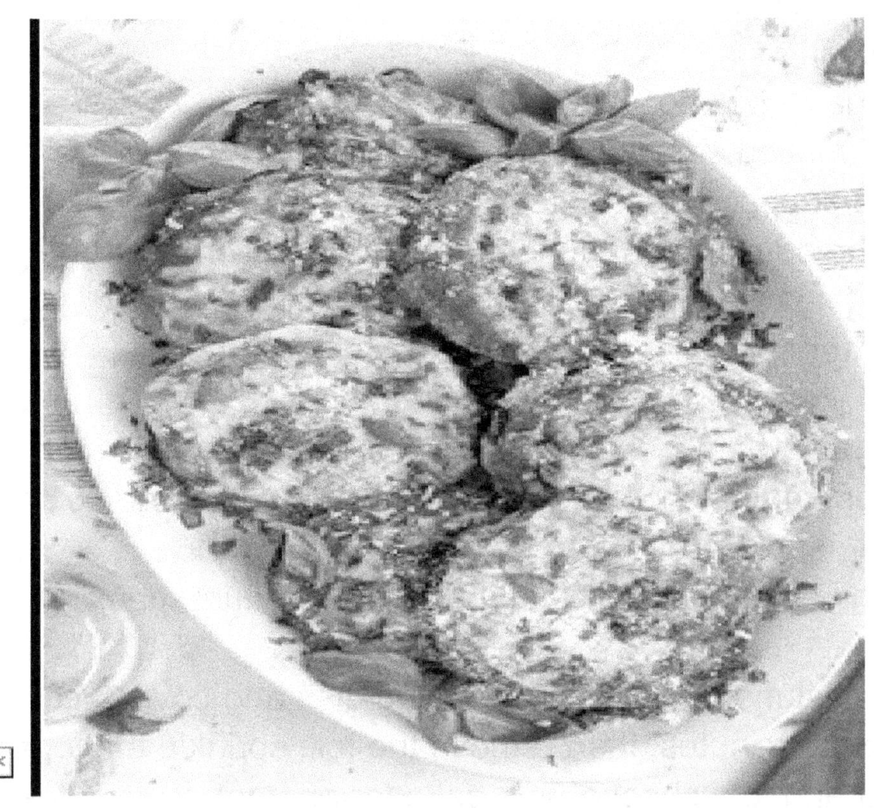

Quinoa Stuffed Bell Peppers
Ingredients:
4 large bell peppers, halved and seeds removed
2 cups cooked quinoa
1 cup black beans, drained and rinsed
1 cup corn kernels, fresh or frozen
1/2 cup diced tomatoes
1/2 cup diced red onion

1/4 cup chopped cilantro
1 tsp chili powder
1 tsp cumin
1/2 tsp garlic powder
1/2 tsp smoked paprika
Salt and pepper to taste
1 cup shredded cheddar cheese (or vegan alternative)
1/4 cup feta cheese (optional)

Instructions:

Preheat your oven to 375°F (190°C).

In a large bowl, mix together the quinoa, black beans, corn, tomatoes, red onion, cilantro, chili powder, cumin, garlic powder, smoked paprika, salt, and pepper.

Fill each bell pepper half with the quinoa mixture, packing it down gently.

Place the stuffed peppers in a baking dish and cover with foil.

Bake for 25 minutes, then remove the foil, sprinkle the tops with cheddar and feta cheese, and bake for another 10 minutes, or until the cheese is melted and bubbly.

Serve hot, garnished with extra cilantro if desired.

Chickpea Tikka Masala

Ingredients:

2 tbsp olive oil
1 large onion, finely chopped
3 cloves garlic, minced
1 tbsp grated ginger
1 can (15 oz) chickpeas, drained and rinsed
1 can (14 oz) diced tomatoes
1 can (14 oz) coconut milk

2 tbsp tomato paste

1 tbsp garam masala

1 tsp turmeric

1 tsp cumin

1/2 tsp chili powder

Salt to taste

Fresh cilantro for garnish

Cooked rice or naan bread for serving

Instructions:

Heat the olive oil in a large pan over medium heat. Add the onion and cook until translucent, about 5 minutes.

Add the garlic and ginger, and cook for another 2 minutes until fragrant.

Stir in the garam masala, turmeric, cumin, and chili powder, and cook for 1 minute.

Add the chickpeas, diced tomatoes, coconut milk, and tomato paste. Stir well to combine.

Bring the mixture to a simmer, reduce the heat to low, and cook for 20 minutes, stirring occasionally.

Season with salt to taste.

Serve the chickpea tikka masala over cooked rice or with naan bread, garnished with fresh cilantro.

Baked Sweet Potato & Black Bean Tacos
Ingredients:

2 large sweet potatoes, peeled and cubed

1 can black beans, drained and rinsed

1 tsp smoked paprika

1/2 tsp ground cumin

1/4 tsp chili flakes (optional)

Salt and pepper to taste
8 gluten-free corn tortillas
1 avocado, sliced
1/4 cup fresh cilantro, chopped
1 lime, cut into wedges
1/2 cup red cabbage, shredded
1/4 cup vegan cheese shreds (optional)
Instructions:
Preheat your oven to 400°F (200°C).
Toss the sweet potato cubes with olive oil, smoked paprika, cumin, chili flakes, salt, and pepper.
Spread the sweet potatoes on a baking sheet and bake for 25 minutes until tender and slightly crispy.
Warm the tortillas in the oven for the last 5 minutes of baking.
Mash the black beans slightly and mix with additional smoked paprika and cumin.
Assemble the tacos by placing a spoonful of black beans on each tortilla, followed by sweet potatoes.
Top with avocado slices, shredded cabbage, cilantro, a squeeze of lime, and vegan cheese if using.
Serve immediately and enjoy!

Cauliflower Rice Alfredo with Gluten-Free Pasta
Ingredients:
1 head of cauliflower, cut into florets
1/2 cup unsweetened almond milk
4 cloves garlic, minced
1 onion, diced
1 tbsp nutritional yeast
1 tbsp olive oil

Salt and pepper to taste
1/4 cup vegan parmesan cheese
8 oz gluten-free pasta of choice
Instructions:
Cook the gluten-free pasta according to package instructions. Drain and set aside.
Steam the cauliflower florets until tender, about 7-10 minutes.
In a pan, sauté the garlic and onion in olive oil until translucent.
In a blender, combine the steamed cauliflower, sautéed garlic and onion, almond milk, nutritional yeast, vegan parmesan, salt, and pepper. Blend until smooth.
Pour the cauliflower Alfredo sauce over the cooked pasta and heat through.
Adjust seasoning as needed and serve hot.
Garnish with extra vegan parmesan and black pepper.

Lentil Shepherd's Pie
Ingredients:
1 cup green lentils, rinsed
2 cups vegetable broth
1 bay leaf
1 tbsp olive oil
1 medium onion, diced
2 carrots, peeled and diced
2 celery stalks, diced
3 cloves garlic, minced
1 tsp dried thyme
1 tbsp tomato paste
1 tbsp gluten-free Worcestershire sauce

1/2 cup frozen peas

1/2 cup frozen corn

Salt and pepper to taste

2 lbs potatoes, peeled and chopped

1/4 cup unsweetened almond milk

2 tbsp vegan butter

Instructions:

Preheat oven to 400°F (200°C).

In a medium pot, combine lentils, vegetable broth, and bay leaf. Bring to a boil, reduce heat, and simmer until lentils are tender, about 25 minutes. Drain any excess liquid and remove bay leaf.

Meanwhile, boil potatoes until tender, about 15 minutes. Drain and mash with almond milk and vegan butter. Season with salt and pepper.

Heat olive oil in a skillet over medium heat. Sauté onion, carrots, celery, and garlic until softened. Stir in thyme, tomato paste, and Worcestershire sauce.

Add cooked lentils, peas, and corn to the skillet. Cook for another 5 minutes. Season with salt and pepper.

Transfer the lentil mixture to a baking dish. Spread mashed potatoes on top.

Bake for 20 minutes or until the top is golden.

Let cool slightly before serving. Enjoy your hearty Lentil Shepherd's Pie!

Stuffed Acorn Squash with Wild Rice Medley
Ingredients:

2 acorn squash, halved and seeds removed

1 cup wild rice blend, rinsed

2 1/4 cups vegetable broth

1 tbsp olive oil
1 small onion, chopped
1 red bell pepper, diced
1 cup mushrooms, sliced
2 cloves garlic, minced
1 tsp dried sage
1/2 cup dried cranberries
1/2 cup pecans, chopped
Salt and pepper to taste

Instructions:

Preheat oven to 375°F (190°C).

Place acorn squash halves cut-side down on a baking sheet. Bake until tender, about 30-35 minutes.

In a medium pot, bring wild rice and vegetable broth to a boil. Reduce heat, cover, and simmer until rice is tender and liquid is absorbed, about 45 minutes.

Heat olive oil in a pan over medium heat. Sauté onion, bell pepper, mushrooms, and garlic until softened.

Stir in cooked wild rice, dried sage, cranberries, and pecans. Season with salt and pepper.

Fill the roasted acorn squash halves with the wild rice mixture.

Return to the oven and bake for an additional 10 minutes.

Serve warm, garnished with fresh herbs if desired.

Eggplant Parmesan with Gluten-Free Bread Crumbs
Ingredients:

2 medium eggplants, sliced into 1/2 inch rounds
Sea salt, for drawing water out of eggplant
2 cups gluten-free bread crumbs
1/2 cup grated Parmesan cheese (or vegan alternative)

1 tsp dried oregano
1 tsp garlic powder
2 eggs, beaten (or flax eggs for vegan option)
2 cups marinara sauce
2 cups shredded mozzarella cheese (or vegan alternative)
Fresh basil leaves for garnish
Olive oil, for frying

Instructions:

Sprinkle sea salt on the eggplant slices and let them sit for 30 minutes to draw out moisture. Rinse with water and pat dry.
Preheat your oven to 375°F (190°C).
Mix bread crumbs, Parmesan cheese, oregano, and garlic powder in a shallow dish.
Dip each eggplant slice into the beaten eggs, then coat with the bread crumb mixture.
Heat olive oil in a pan over medium heat and fry the eggplant slices until golden brown on both sides.
In a baking dish, spread a thin layer of marinara sauce. Layer the fried eggplant slices, top with more sauce, and sprinkle with mozzarella cheese.
Repeat the layering process until all ingredients are used.
Bake for 25-30 minutes until the cheese is bubbly and golden.
Garnish with fresh basil leaves before serving.

Vegetable Stir Fry with Tamari Sauce
Ingredients:
1 tbsp coconut oil
2 cloves garlic, minced
1 inch ginger, grated
1 red bell pepper, sliced

1 yellow bell pepper, sliced

1 cup broccoli florets

1 cup snap peas

1 carrot, julienned

1 zucchini, sliced

1 tbsp tamari sauce

1 tsp sesame oil

1 tsp maple syrup

1 tsp rice vinegar

Sesame seeds for garnish

Cooked rice or rice noodles, for serving

Instructions:

Heat coconut oil in a large wok or frying pan over medium-high heat. Add garlic and ginger, and stir-fry until fragrant.

Add all the vegetables and stir-fry for about 5 minutes, until they are tender but still crisp.

In a small bowl, whisk together tamari sauce, sesame oil, maple syrup, and rice vinegar.

Pour the sauce over the vegetables and stir to coat evenly.

Cook for an additional 2 minutes, allowing the flavors to meld.

Serve hot over rice or rice noodles, garnished with sesame seeds.

Butternut Squash Risotto
Ingredients:

1 medium butternut squash, peeled and cubed

4 cups vegetable broth

1 cup arborio rice

1 small onion, finely chopped

2 cloves garlic, minced

1/2 cup dry white wine

1/4 cup grated Parmesan cheese
2 tbsp olive oil
1 tbsp fresh sage, chopped
Salt and pepper to taste
1/4 cup toasted pine nuts (optional)
Instructions:
In a pot, bring the vegetable broth to a simmer.
In a separate pan, heat the olive oil over medium heat. Add the onion and garlic, and sauté until translucent.
Stir in the arborio rice and cook for 2 minutes until the edges become slightly translucent.
Pour in the white wine and stir until it's mostly absorbed.
Add the butternut squash cubes and a ladle of hot broth. Stir continuously until the broth is absorbed.
Continue adding broth one ladle at a time, allowing each to be absorbed before adding the next.
Cook until the rice is al dente and the squash is tender, about 20 minutes.
Remove from heat, stir in the Parmesan cheese and fresh sage.
Season with salt and pepper.
Serve garnished with toasted pine nuts for added texture and flavor.

Zucchini Noodle Pad Thai
Ingredients:
4 medium zucchinis, spiralized into noodles
1 carrot, julienned
1 red bell pepper, thinly sliced
1/4 cup roasted peanuts, chopped
2 green onions, sliced
1/4 cup fresh cilantro, chopped

1 lime, cut into wedges

2 tbsp coconut oil

For the sauce:

2 tbsp tamarind paste

2 tbsp fish sauce (or soy sauce for a vegan option)

1 tbsp brown sugar

1 tbsp lime juice

1 clove garlic, minced

1 tsp chili flakes (adjust to taste)

Instructions:

In a small bowl, whisk together the tamarind paste, fish sauce, brown sugar, lime juice, minced garlic, and chili flakes to create the Pad Thai sauce.

Heat the coconut oil in a large pan or wok over medium-high heat. Add the spiralized zucchini noodles, carrot, and red bell pepper. Stir-fry for 2-3 minutes until just softened.

Pour the Pad Thai sauce over the vegetables and toss to combine. Cook for an additional 1-2 minutes, allowing the flavors to meld.

Remove from heat and garnish with roasted peanuts, green onions, and fresh cilantro.

Serve with lime wedges on the side for an extra zesty flavor.

Mushroom Spinach Quiche with Almond Flour Crust
Ingredients:
For the crust:

1 1/2 cups almond flour

1/4 cup coconut oil, melted

1/2 tsp sea salt

1 egg

For the filling:

1 tbsp olive oil
1 small onion, diced
2 cups spinach, chopped
1 cup mushrooms, sliced
4 large eggs
1 cup almond milk
1/2 cup feta cheese, crumbled
1/4 tsp nutmeg
Salt and pepper to taste

Instructions:

Preheat the oven to 350°F (175°C).

For the crust: In a bowl, combine almond flour, melted coconut oil, sea salt, and egg until a dough forms. Press the dough into a 9-inch pie dish, forming an even layer on the bottom and sides. Bake for 10 minutes.

For the filling: Heat olive oil in a skillet over medium heat. Sauté onion until translucent, then add mushrooms and cook until they release their moisture. Add spinach and cook until wilted.

In a mixing bowl, whisk together eggs, almond milk, feta cheese, nutmeg, salt, and pepper.

Spread the sautéed vegetables evenly over the baked crust. Pour the egg mixture over the vegetables.

Bake for 35-40 minutes, or until the quiche is set and the top is golden brown.

Let it cool before slicing. Serve warm or at room temperature.

Black Bean & Corn Salad

Ingredients:

1 can black beans, drained and rinsed
1 1/2 cups corn kernels, fresh or frozen (thawed)

1 red bell pepper, diced
1/2 red onion, finely chopped
1/4 cup fresh cilantro, chopped
For the dressing:
3 tbsp olive oil
Juice of 1 lime
1 tsp chili powder
1/2 tsp ground cumin
Salt and pepper to taste
Instructions:
In a large bowl, combine black beans, corn, red bell pepper, red onion, and cilantro.
For the dressing: In a small bowl, whisk together olive oil, lime juice, chili powder, cumin, salt, and pepper.
Pour the dressing over the salad and toss to coat everything evenly.
Refrigerate for at least 30 minutes to allow the flavors to meld.
Serve chilled as a side dish or enjoy it as a light main course.

Roasted Red Pepper Hummus with Veggie Sticks
Ingredients:
1 can (15 oz) chickpeas (garbanzo beans), drained and rinsed
1/2 cup roasted red peppers (from a jar or homemade)
2 cloves garlic
2 tbsp tahini
Juice of 1 lemon
2 tbsp olive oil
Salt and pepper to taste
Fresh parsley or basil for garnish
Assorted veggie sticks (carrots, celery, bell peppers, cucumber) for dipping

Instructions:

In a food processor, combine the chickpeas, roasted red peppers, garlic, tahini, lemon juice, olive oil, salt, and pepper.
Blend until smooth and creamy, adding a splash of water if needed to reach your desired consistency.
Taste and adjust seasoning as necessary.
Serve the roasted red pepper hummus with veggie sticks and garnish with fresh herbs.

Spaghetti Squash with Pesto & Cherry Tomatoes
Ingredients:
1 medium spaghetti squash
1 cup fresh basil leaves
2 cloves garlic
1/4 cup grated Parmesan cheese
1/4 cup pine nuts
1/2 cup extra-virgin olive oil
Salt and pepper to taste
1 cup cherry tomatoes, halved
Fresh mozzarella, diced (optional)
Instructions:
Preheat the oven to 400°F (200°C).
Cut the spaghetti squash in half lengthwise and remove the seeds.
Place the squash halves cut-side down on a baking sheet. Bake for 30-40 minutes or until tender.
While the squash is baking, prepare the pesto. In a food processor, combine basil, garlic, Parmesan cheese, pine nuts, and olive oil. Blend until smooth. Season with salt and pepper.
Once the squash is cooked, use a fork to scrape out the flesh into spaghetti-like strands.

Toss the spaghetti squash with the pesto and cherry tomatoes.
If desired, add diced fresh mozzarella for extra creaminess.
Serve warm and enjoy!

Tofu Veggie Sushi Rolls with Tamari Dip
Ingredients:
4 nori seaweed sheets
1 cup sushi rice (cooked and seasoned with rice vinegar)
1 block firm tofu, sliced into thin strips
1 cucumber, julienned
1 carrot, julienned
1 avocado, sliced
Soy sauce or tamari for dipping
Optional: pickled ginger, wasabi
Instructions:
Lay a nori sheet on a bamboo sushi mat.
Spread a thin layer of sushi rice over the nori, leaving about an inch
at the top.
Arrange tofu, cucumber, carrot, and avocado in a line near the
bottom of the rice.
Roll up the sushi tightly using the bamboo mat. Wet the top edge of
the nori to seal the roll.
Slice the roll into bite-sized pieces.
Serve with soy sauce or tamari for dipping, along with pickled ginger
and wasabi.

Creamy Avocado Soup
Ingredients:
2 ripe avocados
1 cucumber, peeled and chopped

1 cup plain yogurt (or coconut yogurt for vegan)
1 cup vegetable stock
Juice of 1 lime
Handful of fresh cilantro
Salt and pepper to taste
Instructions:
In a blender or food processor, combine peeled avocados, chopped cucumber, yogurt, vegetable stock, lime juice, cilantro, salt, and pepper.
Blend until smooth and creamy.
Taste and adjust seasoning if needed.
Chill the soup in the refrigerator for at least 30 minutes.
Serve cold, garnished with additional chopped avocado, cucumber, and cilantro.

Ratatouille with Gluten-Free Garlic Bread
Ingredients:
1 medium eggplant (aubergine), diced
2 medium zucchinis (courgettes), diced
1 red bell pepper, diced
1 yellow bell pepper, diced
1 large onion, chopped
3 cloves garlic, minced
1 can (14 oz) crushed tomatoes
2 tbsp olive oil
1 tsp dried thyme
1 tsp dried oregano
Salt and pepper to taste
Fresh basil leaves for garnish
For the gluten-free garlic bread:

4 slices of your favorite gluten-free bread
2 tbsp olive oil
2 cloves garlic, minced
1 tbsp fresh parsley, chopped

Instructions:

In a large skillet, heat olive oil over medium heat. Add the onion and garlic, and sauté until softened.

Add the diced eggplant, zucchini, bell peppers, thyme, oregano, salt, and pepper. Cook for about 10 minutes, stirring occasionally.

Pour in the crushed tomatoes and simmer for another 10 minutes until the vegetables are tender.

Adjust seasoning if needed and garnish with fresh basil leaves.

For the gluten-free garlic bread: Preheat the oven to 350°F (175°C).

Mix minced garlic and olive oil in a small bowl.

Brush the garlic oil mixture onto the slices of gluten-free bread.

Bake the bread in the oven for 5-7 minutes until crispy and golden.

Sprinkle with fresh parsley and serve alongside the ratatouille.

Gluten-Free Gnocchi with Spinach Salad
Ingredients:

1 package (16 oz) gluten-free gnocchi
2 cups fresh spinach leaves
1 cup cherry tomatoes, halved
1/4 cup red onion, thinly sliced
1/4 cup pine nuts, toasted
2 tbsp balsamic vinegar
2 tbsp olive oil
Salt and pepper to taste
Grated Parmesan cheese (optional)

Instructions:

Cook the gluten-free gnocchi according to package instructions. Drain and set aside.

In a large bowl, combine fresh spinach, cherry tomatoes, red onion, and toasted pine nuts.

Whisk together balsamic vinegar, olive oil, salt, and pepper to make the dressing.

Toss the cooked gnocchi with the spinach salad and drizzle the dressing over it.

Serve warm or at room temperature, and sprinkle with grated Parmesan cheese if desired.

Vegan Thai Green Curry
Ingredients:
2 colorful bell peppers
1 small eggplant
1 pint grape or cherry tomatoes
3 small zucchini
½ red onion
Extra-virgin olive oil
Kosher salt
Garlic cloves
Crushed red chili flakes
Fresh thyme or rosemary
Balsamic vinegar
Coarse cornmeal (polenta)
Fresh Parmesan cheese (optional)
Butter (optional)
Instructions:
Roasted Vegetables:
Preheat the oven to 400°F (200°C).

Chop up all the vegetables into similar-sized pieces.
Place the chopped veggies in a Pyrex dish.
Drizzle with olive oil and season with salt, pepper, and Italian seasoning.
Mix the veggies until they are well coated.
Roast them in the oven for about 15-20 minutes or until tender. Stir them a few times while they are cooking.

Creamy Polenta:
Bring the water to a boil in a saucepan.
Add the salt.
Whisk in the polenta.
Turn the heat to low and cook until the mixture thickens, stirring often. It will take about 20 minutes.
Remove from heat and stir in butter and cheese (if using).
Serve with the roasted vegetables on top. Sprinkle some Parmesan cheese if desired.

Creamy Polenta with Roasted Vegetables
Ingredients:
1 cup coarse cornmeal (polenta)
6 cups water
2 tsp salt
Butter (optional)
Fresh Parmesan cheese (optional)
Instructions:
Polenta:
Bring the water to a boil in a large pot.
Add the salt.
Whisk in the polenta.

Turn the heat to low and cook until the mixture thickens, stirring often. It will take about 20 minutes.

Remove from heat and stir in butter and cheese (if using).

Roasted Vegetables:

Preheat the oven to 400°F (200°C).

Chop up all the vegetables into similar-sized pieces.

Toss the vegetables with olive oil, salt, and pepper.

Roast them in the oven for about 15-20 minutes or until tender.

Serve the creamy polenta topped with the roasted vegetables.

Moroccan Chickpea Stew

Ingredients:

1 large onion, chopped

3 cloves garlic, minced

2 sweet potatoes, peeled and diced

2 cans (15 oz each) chickpeas (garbanzo beans), drained and rinsed

1 can (28 oz) crushed tomatoes

1 cup vegetable broth

1 tsp ground cumin

1 tsp ground coriander

1/2 tsp ground cinnamon

1/2 tsp ground turmeric

Salt and pepper to taste

Fresh cilantro or parsley for garnish

Cooked quinoa or couscous for serving

Instructions:

In a large pot, sauté the chopped onion and minced garlic in olive oil until softened.

Add the diced sweet potatoes, chickpeas, crushed tomatoes, vegetable broth, and all the spices.

Bring to a simmer and cook for about 20-25 minutes, or until the sweet potatoes are tender.

Season with salt and pepper to taste.

Serve the Moroccan chickpea stew over cooked quinoa or couscous, and garnish with fresh cilantro or parsley.

Stuffed Portobello Mushrooms
Ingredients:
4 large portobello mushrooms
1 cup baby spinach, chopped
1/2 cup ricotta cheese
1 large tomato, thinly sliced
2 cloves garlic, minced
1 tsp Italian seasoning
Salt and pepper to taste
Olive oil
1/2 cup Italian-style breadcrumbs
Instructions:
Preheat the oven to 450°F (230°C).

Remove the stems from the portobello mushrooms and gently scrape out the gills.

Brush the mushroom caps with olive oil and season with salt and pepper.

In a bowl, mix together the chopped spinach, ricotta cheese, minced garlic, and Italian seasoning.

Stuff each mushroom cap with the spinach and ricotta mixture.

Top each stuffed mushroom with tomato slices.

Drizzle olive oil over the mushrooms and sprinkle Italian-style breadcrumbs on top.

Place the stuffed mushrooms on a baking sheet and bake for 15-20 minutes, or until the mushrooms are tender and the breadcrumbs are crispy.
Serve the stuffed portobello mushrooms as an appetizer or alongside a refreshing side salad.

Vegetable Korma with Basmati Rice
Ingredients:
1 large onion, chopped
3 cloves garlic, minced
2 sweet potatoes, peeled and diced
2 cans (15 oz each) chickpeas (garbanzo beans), drained and rinsed
1 can (28 oz) crushed tomatoes
1 cup vegetable broth
1 tsp ground cumin
1 tsp ground coriander
1/2 tsp ground cinnamon
1/2 tsp ground turmeric
Salt and pepper to taste
Fresh cilantro or parsley for garnish
Cooked basmati rice for serving
Instructions:
In a large pot, sauté the chopped onion and minced garlic in olive oil until softened.
Add the diced sweet potatoes, chickpeas, crushed tomatoes, vegetable broth, and all the spices.
Bring to a boil, then lower the heat to a simmer and cook for about 20-25 minutes, or until the sweet potatoes are tender.
Season with salt and pepper to taste.

Serve the vegetable korma over cooked basmati rice, and garnish with fresh cilantro or parsley.

Tomato Basil Soup with Gluten-Free Croutons
Ingredients:
2 tbsp olive oil
1 large onion, chopped
3 cloves garlic, minced
2 cans (28 oz each) whole peeled tomatoes
2 large carrots, peeled and chopped
1 large red bell pepper, chopped
1 tsp dried basil
1/2 tsp dried oregano
Salt and pepper to taste
1 cup vegetable broth
1/2 cup coconut milk (or heavy cream)
Fresh basil leaves for garnish
For the gluten-free croutons:
4 slices of your favorite gluten-free bread
2 tbsp olive oil
1 clove garlic, minced
1 tsp dried basil
Instructions:
In a large pot, heat olive oil over medium heat. Add the chopped onion and minced garlic, and sauté until softened.
Add the whole peeled tomatoes (with their juice), chopped carrots, red bell pepper, dried basil, dried oregano, salt, and pepper.
Pour in the vegetable broth and simmer for about 20-25 minutes, or until the vegetables are tender.
Use an immersion blender to puree the soup until smooth.

Stir in the coconut milk (or heavy cream) and adjust seasoning if needed.

For the gluten-free croutons: Preheat the oven to 375°F (190°C). Cut the gluten-free bread into cubes. Toss the cubes with olive oil, minced garlic, and dried basil. Bake for 10-12 minutes, or until crispy.

Serve the tomato basil soup with the gluten-free croutons on top, and garnish with fresh basil leaves.

Loaded Kimchi Fries

Ingredients:

4 large potatoes, cut into fries

2 tbsp olive oil

Salt and pepper to taste

1 cup kimchi, roughly chopped

1/2 cup cheddar cheese, shredded

1/4 cup green onions, sliced

1/4 cup sour cream

1 tbsp gochujang (Korean chili paste)

1 tsp sesame seeds

1 tsp sesame oil

Instructions:

Preheat your oven to 425°F (220°C). Toss the cut potatoes with olive oil, salt, and pepper.

Spread the fries on a baking sheet in a single layer. Bake for 25-30 minutes until crispy and golden brown.

While the fries are baking, heat sesame oil in a pan over medium heat. Add the kimchi and sauté until it starts to caramelize, about 5 minutes.

Once the fries are done, sprinkle the shredded cheddar cheese over them and return to the oven for a few minutes until the cheese melts.
Top the cheesy fries with the caramelized kimchi, dollops of sour cream, and a drizzle of gochujang.
Garnish with green onions and sesame seeds before serving.

Green Coconut Curry
Ingredients:
1 tbsp coconut oil
1 onion, finely chopped
2 cloves garlic, minced
1 tbsp fresh ginger, grated
2 tbsp green curry paste
1 can (14 oz) coconut milk
1 cup vegetable broth
2 cups mixed vegetables (bell peppers, carrots, peas)
1 block (14 oz) firm tofu, cubed
1 tbsp soy sauce
1 tbsp maple syrup
Juice of 1 lime
Fresh cilantro for garnish
Cooked jasmine rice for serving
Instructions:
Heat coconut oil in a large skillet over medium heat. Add onion, garlic, and ginger, and sauté until the onion is translucent.
Stir in the green curry paste and cook for another minute until fragrant.
Pour in the coconut milk and vegetable broth, and bring the mixture to a simmer.

Add the mixed vegetables and tofu to the skillet. Let it simmer for about 10 minutes until the vegetables are tender.
Stir in soy sauce, maple syrup, and lime juice. Adjust seasoning to taste.
Serve the curry over cooked jasmine rice, garnished with fresh cilantro.

Cauliflower Alfredo with Gluten-Free Pasta
Ingredients:
1 head of cauliflower, cut into florets
4 cups vegetable broth
2 cloves garlic, minced
1 onion, diced
1 tbsp olive oil
1/2 cup nutritional yeast (or Parmesan for non-vegan)
1/2 tsp sea salt
1/4 tsp black pepper
1/4 tsp nutmeg
Gluten-free pasta of your choice
Fresh parsley, chopped (for garnish)
Instructions:
In a large pot, bring the vegetable broth to a boil. Add cauliflower florets and cook until tender, about 7 minutes.
While the cauliflower is cooking, sauté garlic and onion in olive oil in a separate pan until translucent.
Use a slotted spoon to transfer the cooked cauliflower to a blender, adding enough broth to cover it.
Add sautéed garlic and onion, nutritional yeast, salt, pepper, and nutmeg to the blender.

Blend until the mixture is smooth and creamy, adding more broth as needed for desired consistency.

Cook the gluten-free pasta according to package instructions.

Drain the pasta and return it to the pot. Pour the cauliflower Alfredo sauce over the pasta and stir to combine.

Serve hot, garnished with fresh parsley.

Vegetable Stir Fry with Tamari Sauce
Ingredients:

2 tbsp coconut oil

1 red bell pepper, sliced

1 yellow bell pepper, sliced

1 cup broccoli florets

1 cup snap peas

1 carrot, julienned

1 zucchini, sliced

2 tbsp tamari sauce

1 tsp sesame oil

1 tsp maple syrup

1 tsp rice vinegar

Sesame seeds for garnish

Cooked rice or rice noodles, for serving

Instructions:

Heat coconut oil in a large wok or frying pan over medium-high heat.

Add all the vegetables and stir-fry for about 5 minutes, until they are tender but still crisp.

In a small bowl, whisk together tamari sauce, sesame oil, maple syrup, and rice vinegar.

Pour the sauce over the vegetables and toss to coat evenly.

Cook for an additional 2 minutes, allowing the flavors to meld.

Serve hot over rice or rice noodles, garnished with sesame seeds.

Vegetable Paella
Ingredients:
1 cup Arborio rice
2 cups vegetable broth
1/2 cup white wine
1 onion, diced
2 cloves garlic, minced
1 red bell pepper, sliced
1 yellow bell pepper, sliced
1 cup green beans, trimmed and cut into 1-inch pieces
1 cup frozen peas, thawed
1/2 cup artichoke hearts, quartered
1/2 cup cherry tomatoes, halved
1 tsp smoked paprika
1/2 tsp saffron threads
Salt and pepper to taste
Olive oil for cooking
Fresh parsley, chopped (for garnish)
Lemon wedges (for serving)
Instructions:
In a large paella pan or wide skillet, heat olive oil over medium heat.
Add the onion and garlic, and cook until softened.
Stir in the red and yellow bell peppers, green beans, and smoked
paprika. Cook for a few minutes until the vegetables start to soften.
Add the rice and stir to coat with the vegetable mixture. Pour in the
white wine and let it simmer until it has mostly evaporated.

Add the vegetable broth and saffron threads. Season with salt and pepper. Bring to a boil, then reduce the heat to low and simmer for 15 minutes.

Scatter the peas, artichoke hearts, and cherry tomatoes over the top. Do not stir. Continue to cook for another 10 minutes, or until the rice is tender and the liquid has been absorbed.

Remove from heat and let it sit for 5 minutes. Garnish with fresh parsley and serve with lemon wedges.

Miso Glazed Eggplant

Ingredients:

2 large eggplants, halved lengthwise

2 tbsp miso paste

1 tbsp soy sauce

1 tbsp mirin

1 tbsp maple syrup

1 tsp sesame oil

1 clove garlic, minced

1 tsp ginger, grated

Sesame seeds for garnish

Green onions, sliced for garnish

Instructions:

Preheat your oven to 400°F (200°C). Score the cut side of the eggplant halves in a diamond pattern.

In a small bowl, whisk together miso paste, soy sauce, mirin, maple syrup, sesame oil, garlic, and ginger to create the glaze.

Brush the eggplant halves with the miso glaze, making sure to get the glaze into the scored cuts.

Place the eggplant halves on a baking sheet, cut side up, and bake for 25-30 minutes, or until the eggplant is tender and the glaze has caramelized.

Garnish with sesame seeds and green onions before serving.

Late Summer Ratatouille
Ingredients:
2 medium zucchinis, sliced into half-moons
1 large eggplant, cubed
2 bell peppers (one red, one yellow), chopped
3 ripe tomatoes, diced
1 onion, finely chopped
3 cloves garlic, minced
1/4 cup extra virgin olive oil
2 tsp fresh thyme, chopped
1 tsp fresh rosemary, chopped
Salt and pepper to taste
Fresh basil leaves for garnish
Instructions:
Preheat your oven to 375°F (190°C).
In a large baking dish, combine zucchinis, eggplant, bell peppers, tomatoes, onion, and garlic.
Drizzle with olive oil and sprinkle with thyme, rosemary, salt, and pepper. Toss to coat evenly.
Roast in the preheated oven for 35-40 minutes, stirring occasionally, until vegetables are tender and slightly caramelized.
Garnish with fresh basil leaves before serving.
Enjoy this vibrant ratatouille as a main dish or a side to your favorite protein.

Kale Sweet Potato Curry
Ingredients:
1 large sweet potato, peeled and cubed
2 cups kale, stems removed and leaves torn
1 can (14 oz) coconut milk
1 onion, diced
2 cloves garlic, minced
1 tbsp curry powder
1 tsp ground cumin
1/2 tsp ground turmeric
1/2 tsp chili flakes (optional)
1 tbsp coconut oil
Salt to taste
Fresh cilantro and lime wedges for serving
Instructions:
Heat coconut oil in a large pot over medium heat. Add onion and garlic, and sauté until translucent.
Stir in curry powder, cumin, turmeric, and chili flakes, and cook for another minute until fragrant.
Add sweet potato cubes and stir until they are coated with the spices.
Pour in coconut milk and bring the mixture to a gentle simmer. Cover and cook for about 15 minutes, or until the sweet potatoes are almost tender.
Add the kale and continue to simmer for another 5-10 minutes, until the kale is wilted and the sweet potatoes are completely soft.
Season with salt to taste.
Serve hot, garnished with fresh cilantro and lime wedges on the side.

Pumpkin and Sage Gnocchi
Ingredients:
2 cups pumpkin puree
2 1/2 cups all-purpose gluten-free flour, plus extra for dusting
1/2 cup grated Parmesan cheese (optional)
1 large egg
2 tbsp fresh sage, finely chopped
Salt and pepper to taste
4 tbsp unsalted butter
Fresh sage leaves for garnish
Instructions:
In a large bowl, mix together the pumpkin puree, gluten-free flour, Parmesan cheese (if using), egg, chopped sage, salt, and pepper until a dough forms.
Turn the dough out onto a floured surface and divide it into 4 equal parts. Roll each part into a long rope, about 1/2 inch in diameter.
Cut the ropes into 1-inch pieces and press each piece with a fork to create ridges.
Bring a large pot of salted water to a boil. Cook the gnocchi in batches until they float to the surface, then remove with a slotted spoon.
In a large skillet, melt the butter over medium heat. Add the sage leaves and cook until crispy.
Add the cooked gnocchi to the skillet and toss to coat with the sage butter.
Serve hot, garnished with additional sage leaves.

Stuffed Poblano Peppers
Ingredients:
4 poblano peppers, halved and seeds removed

1 cup cooked quinoa
1 can black beans, drained and rinsed
1 cup corn kernels
1/2 cup red onion, finely chopped
1 cup shredded Monterey Jack cheese
1 tsp cumin
1 tsp chili powder
1/2 tsp garlic powder
Salt and pepper to taste
Fresh cilantro for garnish
Lime wedges for serving

Instructions:

Preheat your oven to 375°F (190°C).

In a bowl, combine the cooked quinoa, black beans, corn, red onion, half of the cheese, cumin, chili powder, garlic powder, salt, and pepper.

Stuff each poblano pepper half with the quinoa mixture and place in a baking dish.

Sprinkle the remaining cheese over the top of the stuffed peppers. Cover with foil and bake for 25 minutes. Then, remove the foil and bake for an additional 10 minutes until the cheese is melted and bubbly.

Garnish with fresh cilantro and serve with lime wedges on the side.

Meat Dishes

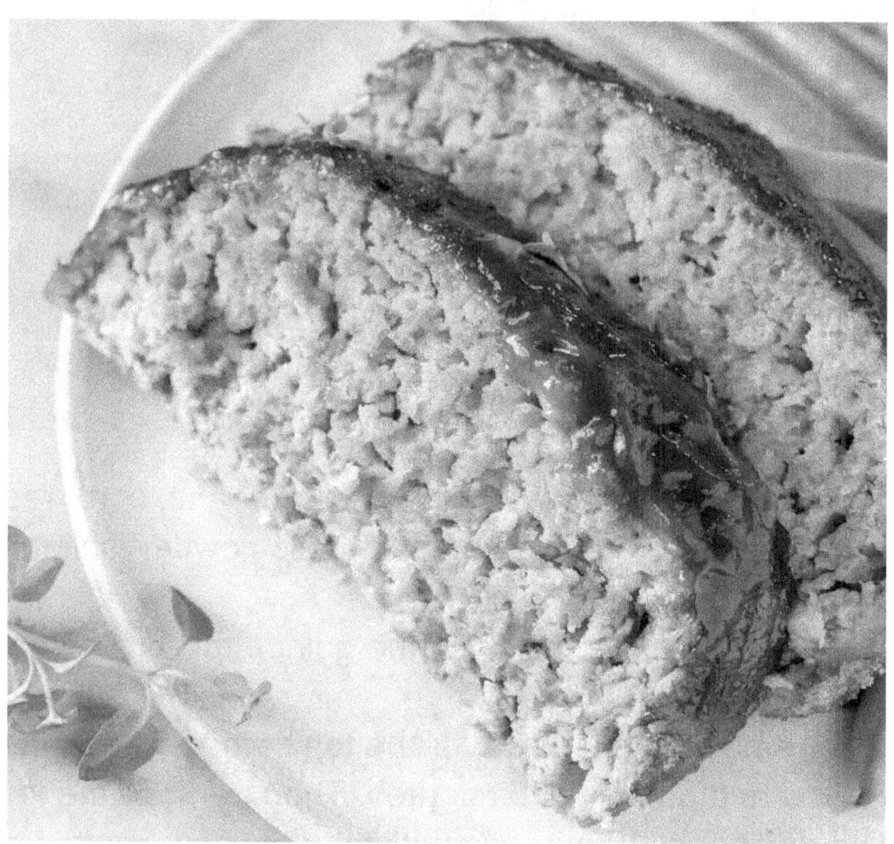

Chicken, Andouille, and Shrimp Jambalaya
Ingredients:
2 tablespoons vegetable oil
1 pound andouille sausage, sliced
2 pounds boneless, skinless chicken thighs, cut into 1-inch cubes
1½ cups chopped onion
1½ cups chopped celery
1½ cups chopped green bell pepper

3 cloves garlic, minced
3 cups long-grain rice
1 (28-ounce) can diced tomatoes
5 cups chicken broth
2 tablespoons chopped fresh thyme
2 fresh bay leaves
1½ pounds large fresh shrimp, peeled and deveined
2 teaspoons kosher salt, divided
1 teaspoon ground black pepper, divided
1 teaspoon smoked paprika
½ teaspoon cayenne pepper
2 tablespoons chopped fresh parsley
Garnish: chopped green onion

Instructions:

Heat oil in a large Dutch oven over medium-high heat. Add sausage and chicken; cook until browned (about 5 minutes).

Add onion, celery, and bell pepper; cook, stirring frequently, until tender (about 3 minutes).

Add garlic and cook for 30 seconds until fragrant.

Stir in rice and toast for about 3 minutes until lightly golden.

Add diced tomatoes and stir until juices are absorbed.

Pour in chicken broth, add thyme and bay leaves. Bring to a boil, then reduce heat to medium-low. Cover and cook for 15 minutes or until rice is tender.

In a medium bowl, combine shrimp, 1 teaspoon salt, ½ teaspoon black pepper, paprika, cayenne, and parsley. Add shrimp to the rice mixture and cook for 2 minutes or until shrimp are pink and firm.

Adjust seasoning with remaining salt and black pepper. Garnish with chopped green onion and serve immediately.

Salmon Niçoise Salad
Ingredients:
1 pound multicolored or red baby potatoes
8 ounces trimmed haricots verts (French green beans)
4 large eggs
2½ teaspoons Dijon mustard
1 teaspoon grated lemon zest, plus 1 Tbsp. fresh lemon juice
1 teaspoon kosher salt, divided
1 teaspoon black pepper, divided
½ cup extra-virgin olive oil, divided
3 tablespoons finely chopped shallot
½ teaspoon honey
1 pound skin-on salmon fillet, any pinbones removed
1 pound mixed lettuces (such as frisée, curly endive, and/or green
leaf lettuce), torn
½ cup pitted Niçoise olives, halved
8 anchovy fillets
⅓ cup torn fresh flat-leaf parsley
Instructions:
Preheat the oven to 400°F.
Boil the potatoes until almost tender (about 10 minutes). Add green
beans and cook until potatoes are tender and green beans are
tender-crisp (about 3 minutes). Transfer to ice water to cool.
Hard boil the eggs (7½ minutes), then transfer to ice water.
Whisk together mustard, lemon zest, ½ teaspoon salt, and ½
teaspoon pepper. Gradually add 6 tablespoons of olive oil to
emulsify.
Drizzle 2 tablespoons of oil onto a baking sheet. Place salmon, skin
side down, on the oiled sheet. Sprinkle with remaining salt and

pepper. Spread 2 tablespoons of mustard mixture evenly over salmon. Bake for 12 minutes or until just cooked through.

Toss lettuces with 3 tablespoons of the mustard-lemon juice dressing. Arrange on a platter or divide among plates.

Top with halved eggs, olives, anchovies, and torn parsley. Place the salmon fillet on top. Drizzle with remaining dressing and serve immediately.

Turkey Meatloaf
Ingredients:
1¼ pounds ground turkey (93% lean)
1 cup Panko breadcrumbs (or regular dry bread crumbs)
½ cup chicken broth
1 large egg
1 tablespoon Worcestershire sauce
2 tablespoons chopped Italian parsley
Salt and black pepper, to taste
1 medium onion, finely chopped
1 red bell pepper, finely chopped
1 carrot, grated
3 garlic cloves, minced
1 tablespoon vegetable or olive oil
Ketchup glaze:
½ cup ketchup
1 tablespoon Worcestershire sauce
1 tablespoon maple syrup (or brown sugar)
Instructions:
Heat vegetable oil in a large skillet over medium-high heat. Sauté onion and bell pepper until softened. Add grated carrot and minced

garlic; cook for another minute. Transfer the mixture to a plate to cool completely.

Preheat the oven to 350°F (175°C) and line a baking sheet with parchment paper.

In a large mixing bowl, combine ground turkey, Panko breadcrumbs, egg, chicken broth, Worcestershire sauce, parsley, salt, pepper, and the cooled vegetable mixture. Mix gently.

Shape the mixture into a 9x3-inch freeform loaf on the prepared baking sheet.

Bake for 30-35 minutes or until the internal temperature reaches 165°F (74°C).

While the meatloaf is baking, prepare the glaze by combining ketchup, Worcestershire sauce, and maple syrup.

Spread the glaze over the cooked meatloaf and broil for 5 minutes until bubbly.

Let it rest for 5 minutes before slicing. Serve and enjoy!

Spicy Shrimp and Sausage Skewers
Ingredients:
1 lb large raw shrimp (16/20 count), peeled and deveined
1 tablespoon Cajun seasoning
2 teaspoons extra-virgin olive oil
7 oz Andouille sausage (or Kielbasa), sliced
Wooden skewers (soaked in water for 30 minutes)
Nonstick cooking spray
Instructions:
Toss the peeled and deveined shrimp with Cajun seasoning and olive oil in a large bowl.
Slice the Andouille sausage to the same thickness as the shrimp.

Skewer the shrimp and sausage alternately onto the soaked wooden skewers.

Preheat the grill to medium-high heat.

Spray both sides of each skewer with nonstick spray and grill for 1-2 minutes per side until the shrimp is opaque.

For impressive grill lines on the sausages, press down with heat-proof grilling tongs while grilling.

Serve the skewers with a creamy, spicy dipping sauce made from mayonnaise, lemon juice, and more Cajun seasoning.

Beef Stroganoff with Mustard and Pickles
Ingredients:
1.5 lbs beef sirloin, thinly sliced
2 tbsp all-purpose flour
4 tbsp unsalted butter
1 large onion, finely chopped
2 cloves garlic, minced
1 cup beef broth
1 tbsp Dijon mustard
1/2 cup sour cream
1/4 cup chopped pickles
Salt and pepper to taste
Chopped parsley for garnish
Cooked egg noodles for serving
Instructions:
Season the beef slices with salt and pepper, then toss them with flour until well coated.

In a large skillet, melt 2 tablespoons of butter over medium-high heat. Add the beef in batches, browning on both sides. Remove the beef and set aside.
In the same skillet, add the remaining butter, onion, and garlic. Cook until the onion is translucent.
Pour in the beef broth and bring to a simmer, scraping up any browned bits from the bottom of the pan.
Stir in the Dijon mustard and sour cream until well combined. Add the browned beef back into the skillet.
Simmer for a few minutes until the beef is cooked through and the sauce has thickened.
Stir in the chopped pickles and season with salt and pepper to taste.
Serve over cooked egg noodles and garnish with chopped parsley.

Pork Tenderloin with Apple Cider and Rosemary
Ingredients:
1 pork tenderloin (about 1 lb)
Salt and pepper
2 tbsp olive oil
2 apples, cored and sliced
1 small onion, sliced
2 cloves garlic, minced
1 cup apple cider
2 sprigs fresh rosemary
1 tbsp apple cider vinegar
1 tbsp honey
Instructions:
Preheat your oven to 375°F (190°C).
Season the pork tenderloin generously with salt and pepper.

Heat olive oil in an oven-proof skillet over medium-high heat. Sear the pork on all sides until golden brown.

Remove the pork and set aside. In the same skillet, add the apples, onion, and garlic. Sauté until slightly softened.

Return the pork to the skillet. Pour in the apple cider, then add the rosemary sprigs.

Transfer the skillet to the oven and roast for 25-30 minutes, or until the pork reaches an internal temperature of 145°F (63°C).

Remove the skillet from the oven and transfer the pork to a cutting board to rest.

Place the skillet back on the stove over medium heat. Add apple cider vinegar and honey, stirring to combine with the pan juices. Cook until the sauce has reduced slightly.

Slice the pork and serve with the apple cider sauce and sautéed apples and onions.

Grilled Tuna Steaks with Mango Avocado Salsa
Ingredients:
4 tuna steaks (about 6 ounces each)
2 tablespoons olive oil
1 tablespoon lime juice
1 tablespoon Cajun seasoning
Salt and pepper to taste
For the Mango Avocado Salsa:
1 ripe mango, diced
1 ripe avocado, diced
1/2 red onion, finely chopped
1 jalapeño, seeded and minced
1/4 cup fresh cilantro, chopped

Juice of 1 lime
Salt to taste
Instructions:
Preheat your grill to high heat.
In a small bowl, whisk together olive oil, lime juice, Cajun seasoning, salt, and pepper.
Brush the tuna steaks on both sides with the mixture.
Grill the tuna steaks for 2-3 minutes per side for medium-rare, or to your desired level of doneness.
While the tuna is grilling, combine mango, avocado, red onion, jalapeño, cilantro, and lime juice in a medium bowl. Season with salt and gently toss to combine.
Serve the grilled tuna steaks topped with the fresh mango avocado salsa.

Chicken Tikka Masala with Coconut Milk
Ingredients:
1.5 pounds chicken breast, cut into bite-sized pieces
1 cup plain yogurt
2 tablespoons lemon juice
2 teaspoons turmeric powder
2 teaspoons garam masala
1 teaspoon cumin
1 teaspoon paprika
Salt to taste
For the Masala Sauce:
1 tablespoon vegetable oil
1 large onion, finely chopped
2 cloves garlic, minced
1 tablespoon grated ginger

1 can (14 ounces) diced tomatoes
1 can (14 ounces) coconut milk
1 teaspoon chili powder
1 teaspoon ground coriander
1 teaspoon garam masala
1/2 teaspoon cayenne pepper
Salt and pepper to taste
Fresh cilantro for garnish

Instructions:

In a bowl, combine yogurt, lemon juice, turmeric, garam masala, cumin, paprika, and salt. Add the chicken pieces and coat well. Marinate for at least 1 hour, preferably overnight.

Preheat your grill or grill pan over medium-high heat. Grill the chicken pieces until cooked through, about 3-4 minutes per side.

For the sauce, heat oil in a large skillet over medium heat. Sauté onion, garlic, and ginger until the onion is translucent.

Add diced tomatoes, coconut milk, chili powder, ground coriander, garam masala, cayenne pepper, salt, and pepper. Bring to a simmer and cook for 10 minutes.

Add the grilled chicken to the sauce and simmer for an additional 5-10 minutes.

Garnish with fresh cilantro and serve with basmati rice or naan bread.

Duck Breast with Spiced Orange Sauce
Ingredients:
2 duck breasts, skin on
Salt and pepper, to taste
1 tsp ground cinnamon

1 tsp ground ginger
1/2 tsp ground cloves
For the Spiced Orange Sauce:
Juice of 2 oranges
Zest of 1 orange
1 tbsp honey
1 star anise
1 cinnamon stick
1/4 cup chicken stock
1 tbsp balsamic vinegar
Salt to taste
Instructions:
Score the duck breast skin in a diamond pattern and season with
salt, pepper, cinnamon, ginger, and cloves.
Heat a skillet over medium heat and place the duck breasts skin side
down. Cook until the skin is crispy and golden, about 6-8 minutes.
Flip the duck breasts and cook for another 4-5 minutes for medium-
rare. Remove and let rest.
For the sauce, discard excess fat from the skillet and add orange
juice, zest, honey, star anise, and cinnamon stick. Bring to a simmer.
Add chicken stock and balsamic vinegar. Simmer until the sauce
reduces by half and thickens slightly. Season with salt.
Slice the duck breasts and serve with the spiced orange sauce
drizzled on top.

Lamb Kofta Kebabs with Fresh Herbs
Ingredients:
1 lb ground lamb
1/4 cup finely chopped fresh parsley
1/4 cup finely chopped fresh mint

1/4 cup finely chopped fresh coriander
1 small onion, grated
2 cloves garlic, minced
1 tsp ground cumin
1/2 tsp ground coriander
1/2 tsp smoked paprika
Salt and pepper, to taste
Olive oil, for brushing

Instructions:

In a large bowl, combine ground lamb, parsley, mint, coriander, onion, garlic, cumin, ground coriander, paprika, salt, and pepper. Mix well.

Divide the mixture into 8-10 portions and shape each around a skewer to form kebabs.

Preheat the grill to medium-high heat. Brush the kebabs with olive oil.

Grill the kebabs, turning occasionally, until browned and cooked through, about 10-12 minutes.

Serve the lamb kofta kebabs hot with a side of tzatziki sauce and warm pita bread.

Fish en Papillote with Citrus and Fennel

Ingredients:

4 white fish fillets (such as cod or halibut, about 6 ounces each)
2 oranges, thinly sliced
1 fennel bulb, thinly sliced
4 sprigs of fresh dill
4 tablespoons of olive oil
Salt and freshly ground black pepper

4 large parchment paper sheets

Instructions:

Preheat your oven to 400°F (200°C).

Season the fish fillets with salt and pepper.

On each parchment paper sheet, place a few slices of orange and a handful of fennel.

Top with a fish fillet, a sprig of dill, and drizzle with 1 tablespoon of olive oil.

Fold the parchment paper over the fish, and crimp the edges to seal, creating a pouch.

Place the pouches on a baking sheet and bake for 12-15 minutes, until the fish is cooked through and flaky.

Carefully open the pouches (watch out for the steam), and serve immediately.

Mediterranean Stuffed Peppers with Ground Turkey

Ingredients:

4 large bell peppers, tops removed and seeded

1 pound ground turkey

1 cup cooked quinoa

1 can (14 ounces) diced tomatoes, drained

1/2 cup crumbled feta cheese

1/4 cup chopped kalamata olives

1/4 cup chopped fresh parsley

2 cloves garlic, minced

1 teaspoon dried oregano

Salt and freshly ground black pepper

Olive oil for drizzling

Instructions:

Preheat your oven to 375°F (190°C).

In a skillet over medium heat, cook the ground turkey until browned. Drain any excess fat.

In a bowl, combine the cooked turkey, quinoa, diced tomatoes, feta cheese, olives, parsley, garlic, and oregano. Season with salt and pepper to taste.

Stuff the mixture into the hollowed-out bell peppers.

Place the stuffed peppers in a baking dish, drizzle with olive oil, and bake for 25-30 minutes, until the peppers are tender and the filling is heated through.

Serve warm, garnished with additional parsley if desired.

Herb-Crusted Chicken Parmesan
Ingredients:
4 boneless, skinless chicken breasts
1 cup gluten-free breadcrumbs
1/2 cup grated Parmesan cheese
1 tbsp Italian seasoning
2 eggs, beaten
1/2 cup all-purpose flour (gluten-free if needed)
2 cups marinara sauce
1 cup shredded mozzarella cheese
1/4 cup fresh basil leaves, chopped
Salt and pepper to taste
Olive oil for frying
Instructions:
Preheat your oven to 375°F (190°C).
Season the chicken breasts with salt and pepper.
Mix breadcrumbs, Parmesan cheese, and Italian seasoning in a shallow dish.

Place the beaten eggs in another dish, and the flour in a third dish.
Dredge each chicken breast in flour, dip into the eggs, then coat with
the breadcrumb mixture.
Heat olive oil in a large skillet over medium-high heat. Add the
chicken and cook until golden brown on both sides.
Transfer the chicken to a baking dish. Spoon marinara sauce over
each breast, then sprinkle with mozzarella cheese.
Bake for 20-25 minutes, until the chicken is cooked through and the
cheese is bubbly and golden.
Garnish with fresh basil before serving.

Maple Glazed Salmon with a Twist of Orange
Ingredients:
4 salmon fillets (about 6 ounces each)
1/4 cup pure maple syrup
2 tbsp soy sauce (gluten-free if needed)
1 tbsp orange zest
1 tbsp fresh orange juice
1 garlic clove, minced
1 tsp Dijon mustard
Salt and pepper to taste
Fresh dill for garnish
Instructions:
Preheat your oven to 400°F (200°C).
In a small bowl, whisk together maple syrup, soy sauce, orange zest,
orange juice, garlic, and Dijon mustard.
Season the salmon fillets with salt and pepper, and place them on a
baking sheet lined with parchment paper.
Spoon the maple-orange glaze over the salmon fillets.

Bake for 12-15 minutes, or until the salmon is cooked through and flakes easily with a fork.

Garnish with fresh dill and serve immediately.

Bacon Wrapped Scallops with Herb Butter

Ingredients:

12 large sea scallops

6 slices of bacon, cut in half

1/4 cup unsalted butter, softened

1 tablespoon fresh parsley, finely chopped

1 teaspoon fresh thyme, finely chopped

1 clove garlic, minced

Salt and freshly ground black pepper

Lemon wedges for serving

Instructions:

Preheat your oven to 425°F (220°C).

Wrap each scallop with a half slice of bacon and secure with a toothpick.

In a small bowl, mix together the butter, parsley, thyme, and garlic. Season with salt and pepper.

Place the bacon-wrapped scallops on a baking sheet and top each with a dollop of the herb butter.

Bake in the preheated oven for 12 to 15 minutes, until the bacon is crispy and the scallops are cooked through.

Serve immediately with lemon wedges on the side.

Grilled Pork Chops with Spicy Peach Salsa

Ingredients:

4 bone-in pork chops, about 1-inch thick

Salt and freshly ground black pepper

Olive oil for brushing

For the Spicy Peach Salsa:

2 ripe peaches, diced

1/2 red onion, finely chopped

1 jalapeño, seeded and minced

1/4 cup fresh cilantro, chopped

Juice of 1 lime

1 tablespoon honey

Salt and a pinch of red pepper flakes

Instructions:

Preheat your grill to medium-high heat.

Season the pork chops with salt and pepper, and brush both sides with olive oil.

Grill the pork chops for 6-8 minutes per side, or until they reach an internal temperature of 145°F (63°C).

While the pork chops are grilling, combine all the ingredients for the peach salsa in a bowl. Season with salt and red pepper flakes to taste.

Let the pork chops rest for 5 minutes after grilling.

Serve the pork chops topped with the spicy peach salsa.

Moroccan Lamb Tagine with Dates and Almonds

Ingredients:

2 lbs lamb shoulder, cut into 2-inch pieces

2 tbsp olive oil

1 large onion, finely chopped

3 cloves garlic, minced

1 tsp ground cumin

1 tsp ground coriander

1/2 tsp ground cinnamon

1/2 tsp ground turmeric

1/4 tsp ground ginger

1/4 tsp cayenne pepper

Salt and black pepper to taste

2 cups beef or lamb stock

1 cup dates, pitted and halved

1/2 cup whole blanched almonds

1 tbsp honey

Fresh cilantro, chopped for garnish

Instructions:

In a large tagine or Dutch oven, heat the olive oil over medium-high heat. Season the lamb with salt and pepper, and brown in batches. Set aside.

In the same tagine, add the onion and garlic, cooking until soft.

Return the lamb to the tagine, and stir in the cumin, coriander, cinnamon, turmeric, ginger, cayenne, salt, and pepper.

Add the stock and bring to a simmer. Cover and cook on low heat for 1.5 hours.

Add the dates, almonds, and honey. Continue to cook, uncovered, for another 30 minutes, or until the lamb is tender and the sauce has thickened.

Garnish with fresh cilantro before serving with couscous or flatbread.

Thai Coconut Curry Shrimp with Pineapple

Ingredients:

1 lb large shrimp, peeled and deveined

1 tbsp vegetable oil

1 small onion, sliced

1 red bell pepper, sliced

2 cloves garlic, minced
1 tbsp fresh ginger, grated
1 can (14 oz) coconut milk
2 tbsp Thai red curry paste
1 tbsp fish sauce
1 tbsp brown sugar
1/2 cup pineapple chunks
Juice of 1 lime
Fresh basil leaves, for garnish
Instructions:
Heat the oil in a large skillet over medium heat. Add the onion and bell pepper, and sauté until softened.
Add the garlic and ginger, and cook for another minute until fragrant.
Stir in the coconut milk, red curry paste, fish sauce, and brown sugar. Bring to a simmer.
Add the shrimp and pineapple chunks to the skillet. Cook for 5-7 minutes, or until the shrimp are pink and cooked through.
Stir in the lime juice and remove from heat.
Serve hot, garnished with fresh basil leaves, over steamed jasmine rice.

Balsamic Glazed Steak Rolls with Asparagus and Red Peppers
Ingredients:
8 thin slices of sirloin or flank steak
16 asparagus spears
1 large red bell pepper, thinly sliced
Salt and pepper, to taste
2 tbsp olive oil
For the Balsamic Glaze:

1/2 cup balsamic vinegar
2 tbsp brown sugar
1 clove garlic, minced
1/4 tsp crushed red pepper flakes

Instructions:

In a small saucepan, combine balsamic vinegar, brown sugar, minced garlic, and red pepper flakes. Bring to a boil, then reduce heat and simmer until the glaze thickens, about 10 minutes.
Season the steak slices with salt and pepper.
Lay out the steak slices and place 2 asparagus spears and a few slices of red pepper on one end of each steak slice.
Roll up the steak around the vegetables and secure with a toothpick.
Heat olive oil in a skillet over medium-high heat. Add the steak rolls, seam-side down, and cook until browned on all sides.
Drizzle the balsamic glaze over the steak rolls and serve immediately.

Spicy Fish Tacos with Cilantro Lime Slaw
Ingredients:
4 white fish fillets (such as cod or tilapia)
1 tbsp chili powder
1 tsp cumin
1/2 tsp cayenne pepper
Salt and pepper, to taste
8 corn tortillas
2 cups shredded cabbage
1/4 cup fresh cilantro, chopped
1 lime, juiced
1/4 cup mayonnaise
1 tbsp sriracha sauce

Instructions:

Preheat the oven to 375°F (190°C).

Season the fish fillets with chili powder, cumin, cayenne pepper, salt, and pepper.

Place the fish on a lined baking sheet and bake for 10-12 minutes until flaky.

In a bowl, mix together the shredded cabbage, cilantro, lime juice, mayonnaise, and sriracha sauce to make the slaw.

Warm the corn tortillas in the oven or on a skillet.

Assemble the tacos by placing a piece of fish on each tortilla, topped with a generous amount of cilantro lime slaw.

Serve with additional lime wedges and enjoy!

Sesame Beef and Broccoli Stir Fry

Ingredients:

1 lb beef sirloin, thinly sliced

2 cups broccoli florets

2 tbsp sesame oil

2 cloves garlic, minced

1 inch ginger, grated

3 tbsp soy sauce

2 tbsp oyster sauce

1 tbsp brown sugar

1 tbsp rice vinegar

1 tsp cornstarch dissolved in 2 tbsp water

Sesame seeds for garnish

Cooked white rice, for serving

Instructions:

In a bowl, whisk together soy sauce, oyster sauce, brown sugar, rice vinegar, and cornstarch mixture. Set aside.

Heat sesame oil in a large skillet or wok over medium-high heat.

Add garlic and ginger, sauté for 30 seconds until fragrant.

Add the beef and stir-fry until browned and nearly cooked through.

Add broccoli and stir-fry for another 2-3 minutes until the vegetables are tender-crisp.

Pour the sauce over the beef and broccoli. Stir well to coat and cook until the sauce has thickened.

Serve over cooked white rice and sprinkle with sesame seeds.

Lemon Herb Roasted Chicken

Ingredients:

4 chicken breasts, bone-in and skin-on

1/4 cup olive oil

Juice and zest of 1 lemon

4 cloves garlic, minced

1 tbsp fresh rosemary, chopped

1 tbsp fresh thyme, chopped

1 tbsp fresh parsley, chopped

Salt and pepper to taste

Lemon slices and additional herbs for garnish

Instructions:

Preheat your oven to 375°F (190°C).

In a bowl, combine olive oil, lemon juice and zest, garlic, rosemary, thyme, parsley, salt, and pepper.

Rub the lemon herb mixture all over the chicken breasts, under the skin, and inside the cavity.

Place the chicken breasts in a roasting pan and arrange lemon slices on top.

Roast in the preheated oven for 35-40 minutes, or until the chicken is cooked through and the skin is golden brown.

Let the chicken rest for 10 minutes before serving. Garnish with additional fresh herbs.

Garlic Mussels in White Wine Sour Cream Sauce
Ingredients:
2 lbs fresh mussels, cleaned and debearded
1 cup sour cream
1/2 cup dry white wine
4 cloves garlic, minced
1 small onion, finely chopped
2 tbsp fresh parsley, chopped
2 tbsp olive oil
Salt and pepper to taste
Crusty bread for serving
Instructions:
In a large pot, heat olive oil over medium heat. Add onions and cook until translucent.

Add garlic and cook for another minute until fragrant.

Pour in the white wine and bring to a simmer. Let it reduce by half.

Stir in the sour cream and season with salt and pepper.

Add the mussels to the pot, cover, and cook for 5-7 minutes until the mussels have opened. Discard any that do not open.

Sprinkle with fresh parsley and give the pot a gentle stir to combine.

Serve hot with crusty bread to soak up the delicious sauce.

Seared Cod with Tomato Caper Sauce
Ingredients:

4 cod fillets (about 6 ounces each)
2 cups cherry tomatoes, halved
1/4 cup capers, drained
3 cloves garlic, minced
1/4 cup fresh basil, chopped
1 lemon, zest and juice
2 tbsp olive oil
Salt and pepper to taste

Instructions:

Season the cod fillets with salt and pepper.

Heat 1 tablespoon of olive oil in a large skillet over medium-high heat.

Add the cod fillets and sear for about 4 minutes on each side, or until golden brown and cooked through.

Remove the cod and set aside. In the same skillet, add the remaining olive oil.

Add garlic and cook for 30 seconds until fragrant.

Stir in the cherry tomatoes and capers, cooking until the tomatoes start to soften.

Add lemon zest and juice, and let the sauce simmer for a couple of minutes.

Return the cod to the skillet, spooning the sauce over the fillets.

Garnish with fresh basil and serve immediately.

Cajun Shrimp with Smoky Garlic Sauce
Ingredients:

1 lb large shrimp, peeled and deveined
2 tbsp Cajun seasoning
1 tsp smoked paprika

4 cloves garlic, minced
2 tbsp olive oil
1/4 cup chicken broth
Juice of 1 lemon
2 tbsp fresh parsley, chopped
Salt to taste

Instructions:

In a bowl, toss the shrimp with Cajun seasoning, smoked paprika, and a pinch of salt.
Heat olive oil in a large skillet over medium-high heat.
Add garlic and sauté until fragrant, about 1 minute.
Add the seasoned shrimp and cook for 2-3 minutes on each side until pink and slightly charred.
Pour in chicken broth and lemon juice, and simmer for another 2 minutes.
Remove from heat, sprinkle with fresh parsley, and serve hot.

Pistachio Crusted Salmon with Spinach and Raisin Salad

Ingredients:

4 salmon fillets (about 6 ounces each)
1/2 cup shelled pistachios, finely chopped
2 tbsp Dijon mustard
2 tbsp honey
Salt and pepper to taste
Olive oil for brushing

For the Salad:

4 cups baby spinach leaves
1/2 cup golden raisins
1/4 cup red onion, thinly sliced
1/4 cup feta cheese, crumbled

2 tbsp balsamic vinegar
1/4 cup extra-virgin olive oil
Salt and pepper to taste
Instructions:
Preheat your oven to 375°F (190°C).
Season the salmon fillets with salt and pepper.
In a small bowl, mix together the Dijon mustard and honey.
Brush the top of each salmon fillet with the mustard mixture.
Press the chopped pistachios onto the mustard layer to form a crust.
Place the salmon fillets on a baking sheet lined with parchment
paper, and brush lightly with olive oil.
Bake for 12-15 minutes, or until the salmon is cooked through and
the crust is golden.
While the salmon is baking, prepare the salad by tossing the
spinach, raisins, red onion, and feta cheese in a large bowl.
Whisk together the balsamic vinegar and olive oil, season with salt
and pepper, and dress the salad.
Serve the pistachio crusted salmon over the spinach and raisin
salad.

Crab Lettuce Wraps with Avocado Cream
Ingredients:
1 lb fresh crab meat, picked over for shells
1 ripe avocado, mashed
1/4 cup sour cream
1 tbsp lime juice
1/2 tsp chili flakes
Salt and pepper to taste
1/4 cup diced red bell pepper
1/4 cup diced cucumber

1/4 cup diced mango
1/4 cup fresh cilantro, chopped
Butter lettuce leaves for wrapping
Instructions:
In a bowl, combine the mashed avocado, sour cream, lime juice, chili
flakes, salt, and pepper to create the avocado cream.
Gently fold in the crab meat, red bell pepper, cucumber, mango, and
cilantro until well combined.
Spoon the crab mixture into the center of each lettuce leaf.
Serve immediately as a refreshing appetizer or light meal.

Creamy Salmon Soup with Dill and Potatoes
Ingredients:
1 lb salmon fillet, skin removed and cut into cubes
2 tbsp olive oil
1 small onion, diced
2 cloves garlic, minced
2 cups vegetable broth
1 cup heavy cream
2 large potatoes, peeled and diced
1/4 cup fresh dill, chopped
Salt and pepper to taste
Lemon wedges for serving
Instructions:
Heat olive oil in a large pot over medium heat. Add onion and garlic,
and sauté until translucent.
Pour in the vegetable broth and bring to a simmer.
Add the diced potatoes and cook until they are tender, about 10
minutes.

Gently place the salmon cubes into the pot and let them cook for about 5 minutes, or until they are just cooked through.

Stir in the heavy cream and fresh dill, and season with salt and pepper to taste. Heat through but do not boil.

Serve hot, garnished with a squeeze of lemon and extra dill if desired.

Shrimp Masala
Ingredients:
1 lb large shrimp, peeled and deveined
2 tbsp vegetable oil
1 large onion, finely chopped
2 cloves garlic, minced
1 inch ginger, grated
1 can (14 oz) diced tomatoes
1 tsp ground cumin
1 tsp ground coriander
1/2 tsp turmeric powder
1/2 tsp garam masala
1/2 tsp red chili powder (adjust to taste)
Salt to taste
Fresh cilantro, for garnish
Lemon wedges, for serving
Instructions:
Heat oil in a large skillet over medium heat. Add onions and sauté until golden brown.

Stir in garlic and ginger, and cook for another minute until fragrant.

Add the diced tomatoes along with cumin, coriander, turmeric, garam masala, red chili powder, and salt. Cook until the tomatoes break down and the oil starts to separate from the masala.

Add the shrimp to the skillet and cook for 5-7 minutes, or until the shrimp are pink and cooked through.
Garnish with chopped cilantro and serve hot with lemon wedges on the side.

Mayo-Free Tuna Salad
Ingredients:
3 cans (5 oz each) tuna in water, drained
1/4 cup extra virgin olive oil
1 tbsp Dijon mustard
Juice of 1 lemon
1/2 cup red onion, finely chopped
1/2 cup celery, finely chopped
1/4 cup fresh parsley, chopped
1/4 cup capers, drained
Salt and pepper to taste
Instructions:
In a large bowl, flake the tuna with a fork.
In a small bowl, whisk together olive oil, lemon juice, Dijon mustard, salt, and pepper to create the dressing.
Add red onion, celery, parsley, and capers to the tuna.
Pour the dressing over the tuna mixture and stir to combine.
Adjust seasoning with additional salt and pepper if needed.
Serve on a bed of greens, in a sandwich, or with your favorite crackers.

Dessert

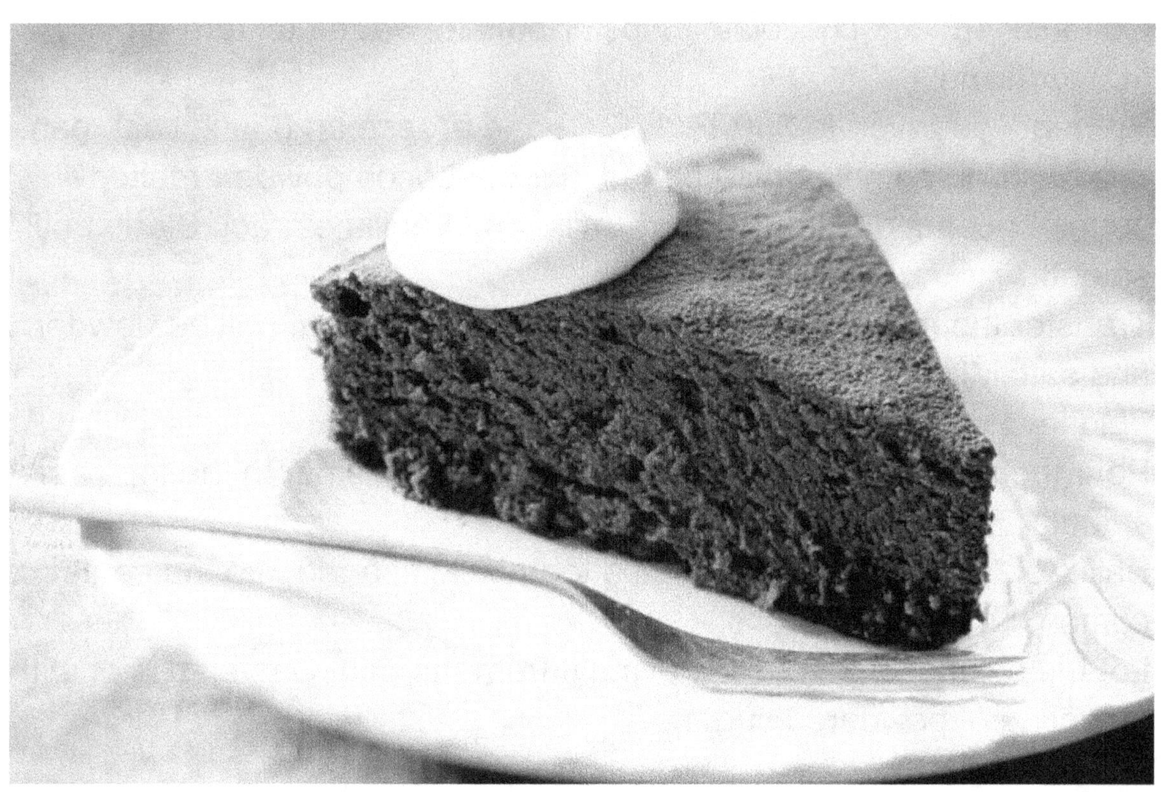

Chocolate Quinoa Cake
Ingredients:
1 cup cooked and cooled quinoa
3/4 cup unsweetened cocoa powder
1/2 cup unsalted butter, melted
1/4 cup coconut oil
3 large eggs
3/4 cup honey or maple syrup
1/2 cup milk of choice
1 tsp vanilla extract

1/2 tsp baking soda
1/2 tsp baking powder
1/4 tsp salt
Optional: 1/2 cup chocolate chips or nuts for added texture
Instructions:
Preheat your oven to 350°F (175°C) and grease an 8-inch cake pan.
In a blender, combine the cooked quinoa, cocoa powder, melted butter, coconut oil, eggs, honey, milk, and vanilla extract. Blend until smooth.
Transfer the mixture to a bowl and add baking soda, baking powder, and salt. Mix until just combined.
Fold in chocolate chips or nuts if using.
Pour the batter into the prepared cake pan and smooth the top with a spatula.
Bake for 35-40 minutes, or until a toothpick inserted into the center comes out clean.
Let the cake cool before removing it from the pan. Serve as is or with a dusting of powdered sugar.

Almond Flour Brownies
Ingredients:
2 cups almond flour
1/2 cup unsweetened cocoa powder
1 tsp baking powder
1/2 tsp salt
3/4 cup unsalted butter, melted
1 cup granulated sugar or coconut sugar
3 large eggs
2 tsp vanilla extract
1/2 cup dark chocolate chips

Instructions:
Preheat your oven to 350°F (175°C) and line an 8x8-inch baking pan with parchment paper.
In a large bowl, whisk together almond flour, cocoa powder, baking powder, and salt.
In another bowl, mix the melted butter and sugar until well combined.
Beat in the eggs one at a time, then stir in the vanilla extract.
Gradually add the dry ingredients to the wet ingredients, mixing until just combined.
Fold in the chocolate chips.
Spread the batter evenly in the prepared baking pan.
Bake for 25-30 minutes, or until the edges are set and the center is still slightly soft.
Allow the brownies to cool in the pan before cutting into squares.

Coconut Macaroons
Ingredients:
3 cups unsweetened shredded coconut
4 large egg whites
1/2 cup honey or maple syrup
1 tsp vanilla extract
1/4 tsp sea salt
Optional: 1/2 cup dark chocolate chips (for dipping)
Instructions:
Preheat your oven to 325°F (165°C) and line a baking sheet with parchment paper.
In a large bowl, whisk the egg whites until frothy. Add the honey, vanilla extract, and sea salt, whisking until well combined.
Fold in the shredded coconut until the mixture is evenly moistened.

Using a spoon or cookie scoop, form the mixture into small mounds on the prepared baking sheet.
Bake for 15-20 minutes, or until the macaroons are golden brown.
Let them cool on the baking sheet for 5 minutes, then transfer to a wire rack to cool completely.
If desired, melt the dark chocolate chips and dip the bottom of each macaroon into the chocolate, then place back on the parchment paper to set.

Lemon Polenta Cake
Ingredients:
1 1/2 cups fine polenta
1 cup almond flour
1/2 cup unsalted butter, softened
3/4 cup granulated sugar
3 large eggs
Zest and juice of 2 lemons
1 tsp baking powder
1/4 tsp salt
Powdered sugar for dusting
Lemon Syrup:
Juice of 1 lemon
1/4 cup granulated sugar
Instructions:
Preheat your oven to 350°F (175°C) and grease a 9-inch round cake pan, lining it with parchment paper.
In a mixing bowl, cream together the butter, sugar, and lemon zest until light and fluffy.
Beat in the eggs, one at a time, then stir in the lemon juice.

In another bowl, whisk together the polenta, almond flour, baking powder, and salt.

Gradually add the dry ingredients to the wet mixture, stirring until just combined.

Pour the batter into the prepared pan and smooth the top with a spatula.

Bake for 35-40 minutes, or until a skewer inserted into the center comes out clean.

While the cake is baking, make the lemon syrup by combining the lemon juice and sugar in a small saucepan over medium heat. Stir until the sugar has dissolved.

Once the cake is done, let it cool for 10 minutes, then poke holes all over the top with a skewer.

Pour the lemon syrup over the cake, allowing it to soak in.

Dust with powdered sugar before serving.

Flourless Peanut Butter Cookies
Ingredients:
1 cup natural peanut butter
3/4 cup coconut sugar
1 large egg
1/2 tsp baking soda
1/2 tsp pure vanilla extract
Pinch of sea salt
Optional: 1/4 cup dark chocolate chips or chopped nuts
Instructions:
Preheat your oven to 350°F (180°C) and line a baking sheet with parchment paper.

In a bowl, mix together the peanut butter, coconut sugar, egg, baking soda, vanilla extract, and salt until well combined.

If using, fold in the chocolate chips or nuts.
Scoop tablespoon-sized balls of dough onto the prepared baking sheet.
Press down each ball with a fork, creating a criss-cross pattern.
Bake for 8-10 minutes, or until the edges are golden brown.
Allow the cookies to cool on the baking sheet for 5 minutes before transferring to a wire rack to cool completely.

Raspberry Frangipane Tart
Ingredients:
1 prebaked 9-inch gluten-free tart shell
1 cup raspberry jam
Frangipane Filling:
1 cup finely ground almonds (almond flour)
1/2 cup granulated sugar
1/2 cup unsalted butter, softened
2 eggs
1 tsp almond extract
1 tbsp gluten-free flour blend
Fresh raspberries for garnish
Instructions:
Preheat your oven to 375°F (190°C).
Spread the raspberry jam evenly over the bottom of the prebaked tart shell.
To make the frangipane filling, beat together the ground almonds, sugar, butter, eggs, almond extract, and gluten-free flour blend until smooth.
Pour the frangipane filling over the raspberry jam layer.

Bake for 30-35 minutes, or until the frangipane is set and golden brown.

Allow the tart to cool completely.

Garnish with fresh raspberries before serving.

Baked Apples with Cinnamon

These baked apples are tender, naturally sweetened, and spiced with cinnamon. They're perfect for a cozy dessert or a healthy snack. Plus, they make your kitchen smell amazing!

Ingredients:

6-7 medium to large apples (a mix of tart like Granny Smith and sweet like Honeycrisp)

2 tablespoons lemon juice

1 tablespoon coconut oil (optional)

2/3 cup coconut sugar (or sub with organic cane sugar or stevia to taste)

1 ½ teaspoons ground cinnamon

3/4 teaspoon fresh grated ginger

A pinch of nutmeg

3 tablespoons cornstarch or arrowroot starch (for thickening the sauce)

3 tablespoons fresh apple juice or water

Optional: Coconut Whipped Cream or Vanilla Bean Coconut Ice Cream for serving

Instructions:

Preheat your oven to 350°F (176°C) and set out a 9x13-inch baking dish.

Peel and core the apples, then quarter them. Thinly slice each quarter lengthwise.

Arrange the apple slices in the baking dish.

In a bowl, mix together lemon juice, coconut oil (if using), coconut sugar, cinnamon, ginger, nutmeg, cornstarch, and apple juice or water.
Pour this mixture over the apple slices in the baking dish.
Cover the dish with foil and bake for 45 minutes. Then uncover and bake for an additional 10 minutes until the apples are tender.
Serve warm with a dollop of Coconut Whipped Cream or Vanilla Bean Coconut Ice Cream.

Sweet & Spicy Pumpkin Seed Brittle
This addictive brittle combines the flavors of maple syrup, sea salt, chili powder, and cayenne. It's crunchy, sweet, and savory—a delightful treat for fall!
Ingredients:
1 cup pumpkin seeds
3/4 cup sunflower seeds
1/3 cup black sesame seeds
2 teaspoons ground cinnamon
1 teaspoon ground ginger
1 teaspoon kosher salt
1/3 cup maple syrup (grade A)
1 1/2 teaspoons vanilla extract
Instructions:
Preheat your oven to 325°F (163°C) and line a rimmed baking sheet with parchment paper.
In a large bowl, combine the pumpkin seeds, sunflower seeds, black sesame seeds, cinnamon, ginger, and salt.
Add the maple syrup and vanilla extract, stirring until well combined.
Spread the mixture evenly onto the prepared baking sheet. Use parchment paper to flatten it to about 1/8 inch thick.

Bake for 25-30 minutes, or until browned.

Remove from the oven and let it cool completely. It will become crisp as it cools.

Break it into small pieces and enjoy the crunchy goodness!

Mango Sticky Rice (Khao Niao Mamuang)

Ingredients:

1 cup Thai sweet sticky rice (also called glutinous or sweet rice) – avoid jasmine rice or basmati rice

1 (14-ounce; 400ml) can full-fat coconut milk, blended well to incorporate fat, divided

1/2 cup sugar (3 1/2 ounces; 100g), divided

Kosher salt

2 teaspoons (6g) cornstarch

2 ripe Ataúlfo mangoes (about 6 ounces or 170g each), peeled, pitted, and sliced

Instructions:

Preparing the Sticky Rice:

Rinse the rice by placing it in a bowl or rice cooker bowl, then swirl your hand to wash.

Repeat rinsing and draining about three to four times until the water is clear.

Soak the rice for at least four hours or overnight in room temperature water for the best results. This softens and enhances the taste absorption of the rice grains.

Once soaked, drain the rice using a mesh sieve and remove excess water.

Spread an even layer of rice on cheesecloth or a clean kitchen cloth to allow steam to pass through effectively.

Wrap and cover the rice with the cloth.
Steam the rice in a rice cooker or steamer for about 20 minutes until tender and cooked.
Making the Coconut Sauce:
In a saucepan, combine half of the blended coconut milk (about 200ml), half of the sugar, a pinch of salt, and cornstarch.
Cook over medium heat, stirring occasionally until the sauce thickens (about 3 minutes).
Turn off the heat and set aside.
Mixing the Sticky Rice and Coconut Sauce:
Once the sticky rice is cooked, pour in 1/4 of the coconut sauce and let it sit for 5 minutes to absorb the flavors.
Serve the sticky rice on a plate with mango slices.
Drizzle the remaining coconut sauce over the sticky rice or serve it on the side.
Enjoy!
Garnish with toasted sesame seeds if desired.
The combination of sweet sticky rice, creamy coconut sauce, and juicy mangoes is simply heavenly!

Chocolate-Dipped Strawberries
Ingredients:
Fresh ripe strawberries (choose firm berries with green leaves intact)
Quality chocolate (white, milk, semi-sweet, dark, or a combination)
Toppings (optional): jimmies, sprinkles, crushed Oreo cookies, graham cracker crumbs, coconut, chopped nuts, or drizzled white chocolate.
Instructions:
Prepare the Strawberries:
Wash the strawberries and allow them to dry thoroughly.

Ensure the berries are at room temperature and dry so the chocolate adheres well.

Melt the Chocolate:

Use a narrow, tall bowl for melting the chocolate (microwave-safe or double boiler).

If using the microwave, heat the chocolate in short increments on 50% power, stirring between each stint.

Dip each strawberry into the melted chocolate, swirling to coat about 3/4 of the berry.

Place the dipped strawberries on parchment paper.

Add Toppings (Optional):

While the chocolate is still wet, sprinkle with toppings like jimmies, crushed Oreos, coconut, or drizzle with white chocolate.

Let Them Set:

Allow the chocolate-covered strawberries to set at room temperature.

Once set, they're ready to enjoy!

Hazelnut Chocolate Mousse

Ingredients:

1 cup milk chocolate, chopped

1 cup heavy whipping cream

1/2 cup toasted hazelnuts, finely chopped (plus extra for garnish)

1 teaspoon vanilla extract

For the Ganache Topping:

1/2 cup heavy cream

1/2 cup milk chocolate, chopped

1 tablespoon hazelnut spread (such as Nutella)

Optional: 1 tablespoon rum

Instructions:
Prepare the Mousse:
Melt the milk chocolate and set aside to cool.
Whip the heavy cream until medium peaks form.
Fold the cooled melted chocolate and finely chopped toasted
hazelnuts into the whipped cream.
Divide the mousse into individual serving cups or glasses.
Make the Ganache Topping:
In a saucepan, heat the heavy cream until it just starts to boil.
Pour the hot cream over the chopped milk chocolate and let it sit for
a minute.
Stir until smooth, then add the hazelnut spread and rum (if using).
Mix well.
Spoon the ganache over the mousse in each cup.
Chill and Garnish:
Refrigerate the mousse for at least 2 hours to set.
Before serving, garnish with additional chopped toasted hazelnuts.

Pavlova with Fresh Berries
Ingredients:
4 large egg whites
1 cup granulated sugar
1 teaspoon white vinegar
1 teaspoon vanilla extract
1 cup heavy whipping cream
Fresh berries (strawberries, blueberries, raspberries)
Raspberry sauce (optional)
Instructions:
Make the Meringue Base:

Preheat the oven to 250°F (120°C) and line a baking sheet with parchment paper.

In a clean, dry bowl, beat the egg whites until stiff peaks form.

Gradually add the sugar, one tablespoon at a time, while continuing to beat until glossy.

Fold in the vinegar and vanilla extract.

Shape the meringue into a round or oval on the prepared baking sheet.

Bake for 1 hour or until crisp on the outside and soft inside. Let it cool completely.

Whip the Cream:

Whip the heavy cream until soft peaks form.

Assemble the Pavlova:

Place the cooled meringue on a serving platter.

Fill the center with whipped cream.

Top with fresh berries (strawberries, blueberries, raspberries).

Drizzle with raspberry sauce if desired.

Serve and Enjoy!

Peanut Butter Chocolate Chip Oat Bars

These Peanut Butter Chocolate Chip Oat Bars are a delicious grab-and-go breakfast or snack. Made in just one bowl and loaded with hearty rolled oats, peanuts, peanut butter, and chocolate chips, these oatmeal bars are everyone's favorite. They're super easy to make too!

Ingredients:

1 cup (2 sticks) butter

1/2 cup brown sugar

1 teaspoon vanilla extract

3 cups old-fashioned oats
1/2 teaspoon ground cinnamon
1/4 teaspoon sea salt
1 1/2 cups chocolate chips
3/4 cup creamy peanut butter

Instructions:

Prepare the Oat Base:

Preheat your oven and coat a 9x9-inch silicone baking pan with cooking spray.

In a large bowl, add rolled oats, chocolate chips, salted peanuts, peanut butter, sweetened condensed milk, and cinnamon. Stir until the ingredients are well combined.

Spread the oat mixture into the prepared pan, pressing it down evenly.

Bake:

Bake for 45 to 50 minutes or until firm to the touch and light brown on the edges.

Cool and Cut:

Cool the bars in the pan, then flip them out onto a cutting board. Cut into squares.

Enjoy!

Store the bars in an airtight container for up to a week or freeze for up to 2 months.

Flourless Chocolate Torte

This Flourless Chocolate Torte is a rich, dark, and creamy dessert that's incredibly decadent. It's a middle ground between a traditional chocolate cake and a molten chocolate lava cake. The subtle almond flavor makes it truly special.

Ingredients:

1 1/2 cups (9 oz) good quality bittersweet or semisweet chocolate, broken into pieces
3/4 cup (1 1/2 sticks) (6 oz) salted butter (or if using unsalted, add 1/4 tsp salt)
6 large eggs, separated (do not mix any yolk with the whites)
3/4 cup (6 oz) sugar
2 tablespoons unsweetened cocoa (you can substitute 1/4 cup (1 oz) of flour if you don't have cocoa and don't mind it not being flourless)

Instructions:

Melt the Chocolate and Butter:

Place the chocolate and butter in a microwave-safe bowl and heat in 30-second increments until both are completely melted and combined.

Whisk the Egg Yolks and Sugar:

In a separate bowl, whisk together egg yolks and half of the sugar until light and fluffy.

Add the chocolate mixture, ground almonds, brandy, and salt. Mix well.

Bake:

Pour the batter into a greased and floured 9-inch springform pan.
Bake at 325°F (163°C) until firm to the touch and light brown on the edges.

Serve and Enjoy!

Dust with confectioner's (powdered) sugar if desired.

Pear and Ginger Crumble

This Pear and Ginger Crumble combines juicy pears with warm ginger and a crunchy crumble topping. It's a comforting dessert that's perfect for fall or any time you're craving something sweet and cozy.

Ingredients:

4-5 ripe pears, peeled, cored, and sliced

Juice of 1 lemon

1 teaspoon grated fresh ginger

1/2 cup granulated sugar (adjust to taste)

1/2 teaspoon ground cinnamon

1/4 teaspoon ground nutmeg

For the Crumble Topping:

1 cup all-purpose flour

1/2 cup rolled oats

1/2 cup brown sugar

1/2 cup unsalted butter, cold and cubed

1/4 cup chopped walnuts or pecans (optional)

Instructions:

Prepare the Pear Filling:

Preheat your oven to 350°F (175°C).

In a bowl, toss the sliced pears with lemon juice, grated ginger, granulated sugar, cinnamon, and nutmeg.

Transfer the pear mixture to a baking dish.

Make the Crumble Topping:

In a separate bowl, combine the flour, rolled oats, brown sugar, and cold cubed butter.

Use your fingers to rub the butter into the dry ingredients until you have a crumbly texture.

Stir in the chopped walnuts or pecans if using.

Assemble and Bake:

Sprinkle the crumble topping evenly over the pear mixture.

Bake for 35-40 minutes or until the topping is golden brown and the pears are tender.

Serve Warm:

Let the crumble cool slightly before serving.

Enjoy with a scoop of vanilla ice cream or a dollop of whipped cream.

Matcha Green Tea Cake

This Matcha Green Tea Cake is a delightful Japanese-inspired dessert. The vibrant green color and earthy matcha flavor make it a unique and delicious treat. The cake layers are light and fluffy, and the matcha frosting adds a creamy touch.

Ingredients:

2 cups all-purpose flour

2 tablespoons matcha green tea powder

1 1/2 teaspoons baking powder

1/2 teaspoon baking soda

1/4 teaspoon salt

1 cup granulated sugar

1/2 cup unsalted butter, softened

2 large eggs

1 cup whole milk

1 teaspoon vanilla extract

For the Matcha Frosting:

1 cup heavy cream

2 tablespoons powdered sugar

1 tablespoon matcha green tea powder

Instructions:

Prepare the Cake Batter:

Preheat your oven to 350°F (175°C) and grease two 8-inch round cake pans.

In a bowl, whisk together the flour, matcha powder, baking powder, baking soda, and salt.
In another bowl, cream the softened butter and granulated sugar until light and fluffy.
Beat in the eggs one at a time, then add the vanilla extract.
Gradually add the dry ingredients to the wet ingredients, alternating with the milk, beginning and ending with the dry ingredients.
Divide the batter evenly between the prepared pans.
Bake and Cool:
Bake for 25-30 minutes or until a toothpick inserted into the center comes out clean.
Let the cakes cool in the pans for 10 minutes, then transfer to wire racks to cool completely.
Make the Matcha Frosting:
Whip the heavy cream with powdered sugar until stiff peaks form.
Gently fold in the matcha powder.
Assemble the Cake:
Place one cake layer on a serving plate.
Spread a layer of matcha frosting over the cake.
Top with the second cake layer and frost the entire cake with the remaining matcha frosting.
Serve and Enjoy!
Garnish with extra matcha powder or edible flowers if desired.

Chocolate Hazelnut Spread (Homemade Nutella)
Ingredients:
1 cup hazelnuts (roasted and peeled)
1/2 cup dark chocolate (70% cocoa), chopped
2 tablespoons cocoa powder

2 tablespoons coconut oil

1/4 teaspoon salt

Optional: 2 tablespoons honey or maple syrup for sweetness

Instructions:

Roast and Peel the Hazelnuts:

Preheat your oven to 350°F (175°C).

Arrange the hazelnuts in a single layer on a baking sheet and roast for about 10 minutes until fragrant.

Let them cool slightly, then rub them in a clean kitchen towel to remove the skins.

Blend the Hazelnuts:

Place the peeled hazelnuts in a food processor or high-speed blender.

Blend for about 3-4 minutes until they turn into a smooth hazelnut butter.

Add the Chocolate and Other Ingredients:

Add the chopped dark chocolate, cocoa powder, coconut oil, and salt to the hazelnut butter.

Blend again until all the ingredients are well combined and the mixture turns into a beautiful chocolate spread.

Adjust Sweetness (Optional):

Taste the spread and add honey or maple syrup if you prefer it sweeter. Blend again to incorporate.

Store and Enjoy:

Transfer the chocolate hazelnut spread to a clean jar.

Store at room temperature for up to a couple of weeks (if it lasts that long!).

Spread it on toast, pancakes, waffles, or enjoy it by the spoonful.

Classic Carrot Cake with Cream Cheese Frosting

Ingredients:

2 cups all-purpose flour
2 teaspoons baking powder
1 teaspoon baking soda
1 teaspoon ground cinnamon
1/2 teaspoon ground nutmeg
1/2 teaspoon salt
4 large eggs
1 1/2 cups granulated sugar
1 cup vegetable oil
2 teaspoons vanilla extract
2 cups grated carrots
1 cup crushed pineapple (drained)
1 cup chopped walnuts or pecans (optional)

For the Cream Cheese Frosting:

8 oz cream cheese, softened
1/2 cup unsalted butter, softened
4 cups powdered sugar
1 teaspoon vanilla extract

Instructions:

Preheat and Prepare:

Preheat your oven to 350°F (175°C) and grease two 9-inch round cake pans.

Mix Dry Ingredients:

In a bowl, whisk together flour, baking powder, baking soda, cinnamon, nutmeg, and salt.

Beat Wet Ingredients:

In another bowl, beat the eggs, sugar, oil, and vanilla extract until well combined.

Combine Wet and Dry Ingredients:

Gradually add the dry ingredients to the wet ingredients, mixing until incorporated.

Fold in the grated carrots, crushed pineapple, and chopped nuts (if using).

Bake:

Divide the batter evenly between the prepared pans.

Bake for 25-30 minutes or until a toothpick inserted into the center comes out clean.

Make Cream Cheese Frosting:

Beat the softened cream cheese and butter until creamy.

Gradually add powdered sugar and vanilla extract, beating until smooth.

Assemble the Cake:

Once the cakes are cool, spread a layer of frosting on top of one cake layer.

Place the second cake layer on top and frost the entire cake.

Decorate with additional chopped nuts or carrot decorations if desired.

Cashew Cream Tart

Ingredients:

For the Crust:

1 1/2 cups almond flour

1/4 cup coconut oil, melted

1 tbsp maple syrup

A pinch of salt

For the Filling:

2 cups raw cashews, soaked overnight and drained

1/2 cup coconut cream

1/4 cup maple syrup

Juice of 1 lemon

1 tsp vanilla extract

For the Topping:

Fresh berries of your choice

Mint leaves for garnish

Instructions:

Prepare the Crust:

Preheat the oven to 350°F (175°C).

Mix almond flour, coconut oil, maple syrup, and salt in a bowl until well combined.

Press the mixture into the bottom and up the sides of a tart pan.

Bake for 12-15 minutes until golden. Allow to cool completely.

Make the Filling:

Blend cashews, coconut cream, maple syrup, lemon juice, and vanilla in a high-speed blender until smooth and creamy.

Pour the filling into the cooled crust and smooth the top with a spatula.

Chill:

Refrigerate the tart for at least 4 hours, or until the filling is set.

Garnish and Serve:

Before serving, top the tart with fresh berries and mint leaves for a burst of color and freshness.

Chocolate Avocado Truffles

Ingredients:

2 ripe avocados, pitted and peeled

1/2 cup unsweetened cocoa powder, plus extra for rolling

1/2 cup dark chocolate chips, melted

1/4 cup honey or agave syrup

1 tsp vanilla extract

A pinch of sea salt

Instructions:

Prepare the Truffle Mixture:

In a food processor, blend the avocado until smooth.

Add the cocoa powder, melted chocolate, honey, vanilla extract, and sea salt. Blend until you have a homogeneous mixture.

Chill:

Transfer the mixture to a bowl and refrigerate for about 30 minutes, or until it's firm enough to handle.

Form the Truffles:

Once chilled, use a spoon to scoop out balls of the mixture.

Roll each ball in your hands and then roll in cocoa powder to coat.

Serve or Store:

Enjoy immediately or store in the refrigerator for up to a week.

Sauces and Dressings

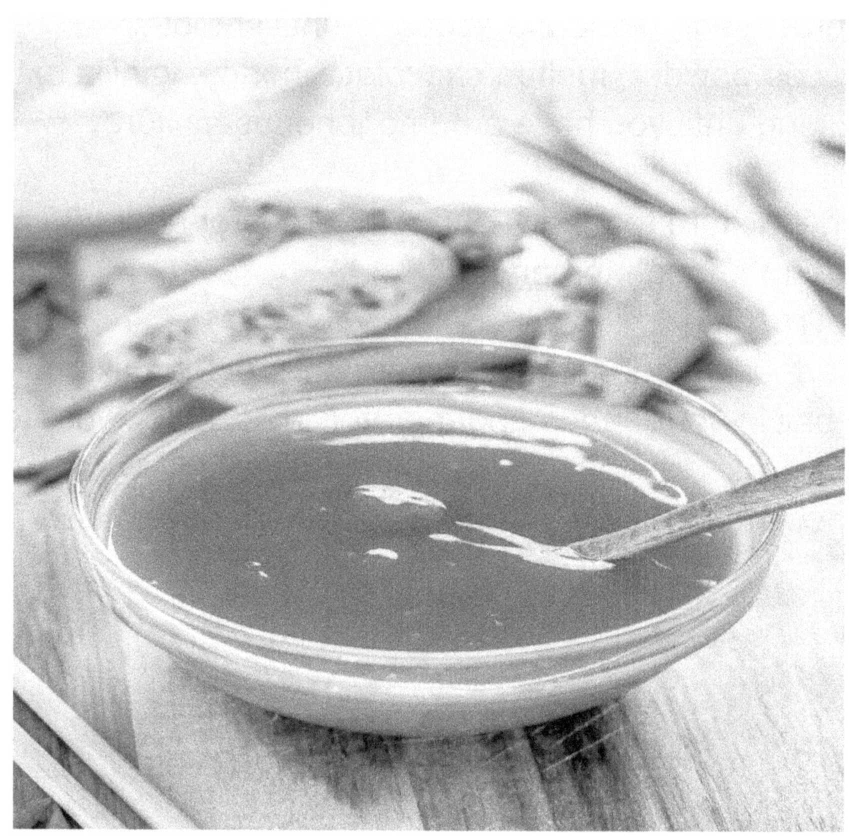

Sweet & Sour Cream Sauce
Ingredients:
1 cup pineapple juice
2 tablespoons tamari sauce (gluten-free soy sauce)
2 tablespoons rice vinegar
2 tablespoons honey or maple syrup
1 teaspoon arrowroot powder (or cornstarch)
Pinch of red pepper flakes (optional, for heat)

Instructions:

In a small bowl, mix the pineapple juice, tamari sauce, rice vinegar, and honey (or maple syrup).

In a separate bowl, dissolve the arrowroot powder in a tablespoon of cold water.

Heat a saucepan over medium heat and pour in the pineapple mixture.

Stir in the dissolved arrowroot powder to thicken the sauce.

Add a pinch of red pepper flakes if you like it spicy.

Simmer for a few minutes until the sauce thickens and becomes glossy.

Taste and adjust the sweetness or tanginess as desired.

Serve over grilled chicken, tofu, or stir-fried vegetables.

Vegan Cashew Cream Sauce

Ingredients:

1 cup raw cashews (soaked in water for at least 2 hours or overnight)

1 cup purified water

Juice of 1 lemon

Salt and pepper to taste

Instructions:

Drain and rinse the soaked cashews.

In a blender or food processor, combine the cashews, purified water, and lemon juice.

Blend until smooth and creamy. Adjust the water if needed to achieve the desired consistency.

Season with salt and pepper to taste.

Use the cashew cream sauce as a base for pasta dishes, as a dip, or drizzle it over roasted vegetables.

Vegan Dulce de Leche
Ingredients:
1 can (13.5 oz) full-fat coconut milk
1/2 cup coconut sugar
1/2 teaspoon vanilla extract
Pinch of sea salt
Instructions:
Pour the coconut milk into a saucepan and add the coconut sugar.
Stir over medium heat until the sugar has dissolved.
Once the mixture starts to boil, reduce the heat to low and simmer.
Stir frequently for about 30-40 minutes, or until the mixture thickens
and turns a caramel color.
Remove from heat and stir in the vanilla extract and a pinch of sea
salt.
Allow it to cool before using. It will continue to thicken as it cools.
Store in a jar in the refrigerator. Use it as a spread, drizzle, or
sweetener for desserts and beverages.
Roasted Red Pepper Sauce
Ingredients:
4 large red bell peppers
1/4 cup toasted almonds or walnuts
1 small ripe plum tomato, chopped
2 tablespoons extra virgin olive oil
1 tablespoon red wine vinegar
1 garlic clove, minced
Salt and pepper to taste
Optional: 1/4 cup heavy cream or non-dairy milk for creaminess
Instructions:

Preheat your oven to 450°F (232°C). Place the red peppers on a baking sheet and roast for 20-25 minutes, turning occasionally, until the skins are charred.

Remove from the oven and place in a bowl. Cover with plastic wrap and let them steam for 10 minutes.

Peel the skins off the peppers and remove the seeds.

In a blender, combine the roasted peppers, toasted nuts, tomato, olive oil, red wine vinegar, and minced garlic.

Blend until smooth. If you want a creamier sauce, add heavy cream or non-dairy milk and blend again.

Season with salt and pepper to taste.

Serve with pasta, grilled meats, or as a dip for vegetables.

Vegan Garlic Pasta Sauce
Ingredients:
1 cup raw cashews, soaked for 4 hours
2 tablespoons nutritional yeast
4 cloves garlic, minced
2 tablespoons olive oil
1 tablespoon lemon juice
1/2 teaspoon onion powder
Salt and pepper to taste
1/2 cup water (or as needed for consistency)
Instructions:
Begin by soaking the cashews in water for at least 4 hours, or overnight for best results.

Drain and rinse the cashews, then place them in a blender.

Add the nutritional yeast, minced garlic, olive oil, lemon juice, onion powder, salt, and pepper.

Blend on high until smooth and creamy, adding water as needed to reach your desired consistency.

Taste and adjust seasoning if necessary.

Serve over your favorite gluten-free pasta and garnish with fresh herbs.

Pesto Sauce

Ingredients:

2 cups fresh basil leaves

1/2 cup pine nuts, toasted

2 cloves garlic

1/2 cup extra-virgin olive oil

1/4 cup nutritional yeast

Juice of 1/2 lemon

Salt and pepper to taste

Instructions:

In a food processor, combine the basil leaves, toasted pine nuts, and garlic.

Pulse until coarsely chopped.

With the processor running, slowly pour in the olive oil and continue to process until fully incorporated and smooth.

Add the nutritional yeast, lemon juice, salt, and pepper.

Pulse again to combine all the ingredients.

Taste and adjust the seasoning as needed.

Use immediately or store in an airtight container in the refrigerator.

Gluten-Free Roux Recipe

Ingredients:

1/4 cup unsalted butter or olive oil for a dairy-free version

1/4 cup gluten-free all-purpose flour blend (ensure it's xanthan gum-free)

1/2 teaspoon garlic powder (optional for added flavor)
1/2 teaspoon onion powder (optional for added flavor)
Salt and pepper to taste
Instructions:
In a small saucepan, melt the butter over medium heat. If you're
using olive oil, heat it until it's warm but not smoking.
Slowly whisk in the gluten-free flour blend until it's fully incorporated
with the fat. If you're adding garlic and onion powder, do so now.
Continue to cook the mixture, whisking constantly, for about 2-3
minutes. This will help cook out the raw flavor of the flour.
Once the roux has turned a light golden color and has a nutty aroma,
remove it from the heat. Season with salt and pepper to your liking.
Your gluten-free roux is now ready to use! It can thicken
approximately one cup of liquid. If you need more, simply scale up
the recipe keeping the fat-to-flour ratio equal.

Honey Mustard Vinaigrette
Ingredients:
2 tablespoons Dijon mustard
2 tablespoons honey
3 tablespoons apple cider vinegar
1/4 cup extra-virgin olive oil
Salt and pepper to taste
Instructions:
In a small bowl, whisk together the Dijon mustard and honey until
well combined.
Gradually add the apple cider vinegar while continuing to whisk.
Slowly drizzle in the olive oil, whisking constantly to emulsify the
dressing.

Season with salt and pepper to taste.
Taste and adjust the sweetness or tanginess by adding more honey or vinegar if desired.
Drizzle over mixed greens, grilled chicken, or roasted vegetables.

Balsamic Fig Dressing
Ingredients:
6 dried figs
1/2 cup balsamic vinegar
1/4 cup extra-virgin olive oil
1 tablespoon honey
Salt and pepper to taste
Instructions:
In a small saucepan, combine the dried figs and balsamic vinegar.
Simmer over low heat for about 10 minutes, or until the figs are softened.
Remove from heat and let it cool slightly.
Transfer the figs and vinegar to a blender or food processor.
Add the olive oil, honey, salt, and pepper.
Blend until smooth and well combined.
Taste and adjust the sweetness or acidity as needed.
Drizzle this flavorful dressing over salads with goat cheese, arugula, and toasted walnuts.

Asian Sesame Dressing
Ingredients:
2 tablespoons toasted sesame oil
2 tablespoons rice vinegar
1 tablespoon soy sauce (or tamari for gluten-free)
1 teaspoon grated fresh ginger

1 clove garlic, minced
1 teaspoon honey or maple syrup (adjust to taste)
1 green onion, finely chopped
Optional: 1 teaspoon sesame seeds for garnish
Instructions:
In a small bowl, whisk together the toasted sesame oil, rice vinegar, soy sauce, grated ginger, minced garlic, and honey (or maple syrup).
Taste the dressing and adjust the sweetness or saltiness as desired.
Add the finely chopped green onion and mix well.
Let the flavors meld for at least 15 minutes before serving.
Drizzle this Asian sesame dressing over salads, steamed vegetables, or use it as a marinade for grilled tofu or chicken.

Maple Dijon Dressing
Ingredients:
2 tablespoons Dijon mustard
2 tablespoons pure maple syrup
3 tablespoons apple cider vinegar
1/4 cup extra-virgin olive oil
Salt and pepper to taste
Instructions:
In a small bowl, whisk together the Dijon mustard and maple syrup until well combined.
Gradually add the apple cider vinegar while continuing to whisk.
Slowly drizzle in the olive oil, whisking constantly to emulsify the dressing.
Season with salt and pepper to taste.
Taste and adjust the sweetness or tanginess by adding more maple syrup or vinegar if desired.

This Maple Dijon dressing pairs beautifully with mixed greens, roasted vegetables, or grain salads.

Lemon Herb Dressing
Ingredients:
Juice of 1 lemon
Zest of 1 lemon
1/4 cup extra-virgin olive oil
2 tablespoons fresh parsley, finely chopped
1 tablespoon fresh basil, finely chopped
1 clove garlic, minced
Salt and pepper to taste
Instructions:
In a small bowl, whisk together the lemon juice, lemon zest, and minced garlic.
Slowly drizzle in the olive oil while continuing to whisk.
Add the chopped parsley and basil, and season with salt and pepper.
Taste and adjust the flavors as needed.
Let the dressing sit for a few minutes to allow the herbs to infuse.
Drizzle over salads, grilled chicken, or roasted vegetables.

Avocado Crema
Ingredients:
1 ripe avocado
Juice of 1 lime
1/4 cup plain Greek yogurt (or dairy-free yogurt for a vegan version)
1 clove garlic, minced
Salt and pepper to taste

Optional: A pinch of cayenne pepper for some heat
Instructions:
Cut the avocado in half, remove the pit, and scoop out the flesh.
Mash the avocado in a bowl until smooth.
Add the lime juice, minced garlic, and Greek yogurt. Mix well.
Season with salt, pepper, and a pinch of cayenne if desired.
Adjust the consistency by adding more yogurt or lime juice.
Use this creamy avocado crema as a topping for tacos, grilled fish, or as a dip for vegetable sticks.

Appendix

Conversion of the Units of Measurement

Volume Conversions:
1 tablespoon (tbsp) = 3 teaspoons (tsp)
1 fluid ounce (fl oz) = 2 tablespoons
1 cup = 8 fluid ounces
1 pint (pt) = 2 cups
1 quart (qt) = 2 pints
1 gallon (gal) = 4 quarts

Weight Conversions:
1 ounce (oz) = 28.35 grams (g)
1 pound (lb) = 16 ounces

Dry Ingredient Conversions:
1 cup all-purpose flour = 120 grams
1 cup granulated sugar = 200 grams
1 cup butter = 227 grams

The Dirty Dozen and Clean Fifteen

The "Dirty Dozen" and "Clean fifteen" are lists published annually by the Environmental Working Group (EWG) to inform consumers about fruits and vegetables with the highest and lowest pesticide residues, respectively.

The Dirty Dozen for 2024
Strawberries: Often top the list due to the high number of pesticides used in their cultivation.
Spinach: Tends to absorb pesticides and chemicals from the soil and water.
Kale, Collard, and Mustard Greens: Leafy greens with a large surface area that can retain pesticides.
Grapes: Thin-skinned and often treated with multiple pesticides.
Peaches: Soft skin can absorb pesticides, which are used to fend off insects and disease.
Pears: Similar to peaches, pears have soft skin and may be treated with several pesticides.
Nectarines: Their delicate skin and susceptibility to pests make them prone to pesticide use.
Apples: A popular fruit that is often treated with pesticides to maintain year-round availability.
Bell & Hot Peppers: Their thin skin doesn't offer much protection from pesticide sprays.
Cherries: Like other soft fruits, cherries may be sprayed multiple times before harvest.
Blueberries: Small and quick to spoil, they are often treated with pesticides to extend shelf life.
Green Beans: May be treated with pesticides to protect against insects and diseases.

The Clean 15 for 2024

Avocados: Thick skin protects the fruit from pesticide residue.

Sweet Corn: Generally has low pesticide residue; note that some may be from genetically modified seeds.

Pineapple: Hard outer shell provides protection from pesticide absorption.

Onions: Less susceptible to pests and thus require fewer pesticides.

Papaya: Some are GMO but generally have low pesticide residue.

Sweet Peas (Frozen): Typically have low levels of pesticide residue.

Asparagus: Fewer pest threats mean fewer pesticides are needed.

Honeydew Melon: Thick rind keeps pesticide residue out of the flesh.

Kiwi: Its skin provides a barrier to pesticides.

Cabbage: Does not attract many pests, so it's not heavily sprayed.

Mushrooms: Grown in controlled environments and thus less likely to need pesticides.

Mangoes: Thick skin protects the fruit from most pesticide residues.

Watermelon: Like other melons, its thick rind prevents pesticide residue in the flesh.

Carrots: Generally have low pesticide residue.

Sweet Potatoes: Less prone to pests and diseases, so they require fewer pesticides.

For gluten-free consumers, the relevance of these lists extends beyond just pesticide exposure. Gluten-free diets often rely heavily on fruits and vegetables as staple foods. Therefore, understanding which items have higher pesticide residues can guide safer food choices, especially for those with heightened food sensitivities or autoimmune conditions like celiac disease.

www.ingramcontent.com/pod-product-compliance
Lightning Source LLC
Chambersburg PA
CBHW081514250726
48659CB00009B/2804